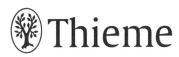

Practical Breast Pathology
2nd edition

Tibor Tot, MD
Associate Professor
Department of Pathology and Clinical Cytology
Falun Central Hospital
Falun, Sweden

László Tabár, MD
Professor Emeritus
Department of Mammography
Falun Central Hospital
Falun, Sweden

Peter B. Dean, MD
Professor Emeritus
Department of Diagnostic Radiology
University Central Hospital
Turku, Finland

Former Director of Breast Imaging
Turku University Hospital
Turku, Finland

521 illustrations

Thieme
Stuttgart · New York · Delhi · Rio

Library of Congress Cataloging-in-Publication Data is available from the publisher.

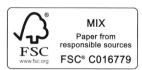

© 2014 Georg Thieme Verlag KG
Thieme Publishers Stuttgart
Rüdigerstrasse 14, 70469 Stuttgart, Germany
+49 [0]711 8931 421
customerservice@thieme.de

Thieme Publishers New York
333 Seventh Avenue, New York
NY 10001 USA, 1-800-782-3488
customerservice@thieme.com

Thieme Publishers Delhi
A-12, Second Floor, Sector -2, Noida -201301
Uttar Pradesh, India, +91 120 45 566 00
customerservice@thieme.in

Thieme Publishers Rio, Thieme Publicações Ltda.
Argentina Building 16th floor, Ala A, 228 Praia do Botafogo
Rio de Janeiro 22250-040 Brazil, +55 21 3736-3631

Cover design: Thieme Publishing Group
Typesetting by: Thomson Digital, NSEZ, Noida, India
Printed by: Replika Press Pvt Ltd, India

ISBN 978-3-13-129432-6   1 2 3 4 5

Also available as an e-book:
eISBN 978-3-13-160782-9

This book is dedicated to Mária, Viktória, and Kirsti.

Preface to the Second Edition

The rapid developments in breast imaging and molecular pathology during the last decade have opened new perspectives in diagnosing breast diseases and increased the responsibilities of both the individual members of the breast team and the team as a whole. Interdisciplinary diagnosis advocated by the authors in the first edition of this book has become the new gold standard in diagnosing breast carcinoma. Understanding the morphology of normal and pathologically altered breast tissue is still the most important basis for making proper diagnosis, but new discoveries and changing views continuously enrich our knowledge and influence the practice in many institutions. This progress motivated the authors to update the content of this monograph. The authors intended to keep the original approach of the first edition to provide the necessary information for the non-pathologist, without details relevant only for pathologists, but at the same time aimed to provide essential molecular biological facts and a theoretic foundation, thus advancing our understanding of the natural history of breast lesions. A substantial part of the material presented in the second edition of the book is based on the authors' own studies and theories published during the last decade and also on their experience with multimodality radiology (digital mammography, ultrasonography, and magnetic resonance imaging) and 2D and 3D large-format histopathology correlation. The authors hope that breast radiologists, pathologists, and clinicians will find inspiration in the presented content and elements to implement into their everyday cooperation within the breast team.

Tibor Tot
László Tabár
Peter B. Dean

Preface to the First Edition

Radiologists, surgeons, oncologists, and other specialists working with diseases of the breast can perform far more effectively when they have a firm understanding of breast pathology. Fortunately, it is only the pathologist who needs to make histologic diagnoses. This book strives to provide information which the non-pathologist needs to know and the pathologist should provide about breast diseases, without burdening the reader with details relevant only to the pathologist. Our approach emphasizes mammographic–pathologic correlation, explaining why two radiologists have joined a pathologist to write this book.

The material presented in this book has come exclusively from the Departments of Pathology and Mammography of the Central Hospital of Falun, Sweden, with patient follow-up exceeding 25 years. A collection of more than 3,000 breast cancer cases with mammographic, specimen radiology, and large-section pathology correlation has been the source of our material, which includes several hundred cases with additional thick-section pathology.

Interdisciplinary diagnosis and treatment of breast diseases is slowly but irrevocably becoming accepted as the new golden standard for patient care. It requires an additional investment of time and effort, which is soon repaid by smoother delivery of care and far fewer iatrogenic complications. Interdisciplinary breast teamwork is a dynamic and demanding process, the ultimate reward of which is a significant improvement in patient care. This book has been written to assist in the implementation of interdisciplinary breast teamwork, to help the radiologist and pathologist communicate with each other, and to provide a framework for everyday cooperation within the breast team.

Tibor Tot
László Tabár
Peter B. Dean

Acknowledgments

The authors thank all the members of the breast team in Dalarna County and all the personnel of the Departments of Mammography, Surgery, and Pathology for their valued support.

Contents

Chapter 1

Normal Breast Tissue or Fibrocystic Change?

The mammary gland, like all glandular organs, consists of parenchyma and stroma. The parenchyma contains ducts (**Figs. 1.1** and **1.2**, thick-section image) and lobules (**Fig. 1.3**), which are separated from the stroma by a continuous basement membrane (**Fig. 1.4**, Sirius Red staining). The entire parenchyma (with the exception of the terminal parts of the lactiferous ducts covered by squamous epithelium) consists of a single inner layer of epithelial cells and an outer layer of myoepithelium (**Fig. 1.5**, α smooth-muscle actin stain). Only the epithelial cells contain estrogen and progesterone receptors in their nuclei (**Fig. 1.6**).

The stroma consists of fibrous tissue and adipose tissue containing lymph vessels, blood vessels, and nerves. More specialized within the lobules and surrounding the ducts, the stroma can be divided into intralobular (mucin-rich, "active") and interlobular stroma (see **Fig. 1.19**, Alcian Blue staining).

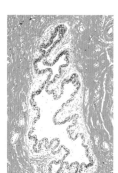

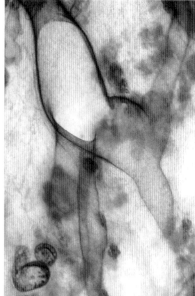

Fig. 1.1   **Fig. 1.2**

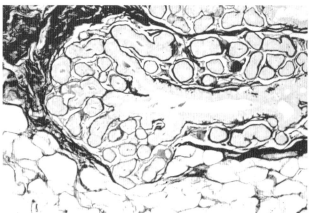

Fig. 1.3

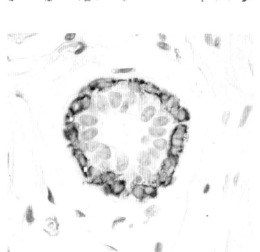

Fig. 1.4

The nipple is the origin of 15 to 25 lactiferous ducts, which branch into segmental, subsegmental, and terminal ducts that, with the associated lobules and stroma, constitute 15 to 25 lobes. The lobes are individual units with only exceptionally rare anastomotic interconnections. The size and shape of the lobes vary greatly, and their interrelation is complex. This has been demonstrated by filling the lobes of breasts from cadavers with colored hot wax (**Fig. 1.7**; *On the Anatomy of the Breast* by Cooper AP). Individual lobes, their ducts and lobules are routinely visualized using contrast medium in patients with serous or bloody nipple discharge (**Fig. 1.8**, galactography image). Structures belonging to a segmental branch of the ductal tree constitute an anatomical segment of the breast. The terminal duct and the associated lobule are collectively referred to as the terminal ductal-lobular unit (TDLU), which is the most important functional unit and the place of origin of many pathological processes in the breast (**Figs. 1.9** and **1.10**). Malignancy may, however, develop in any part of a sick lobe.

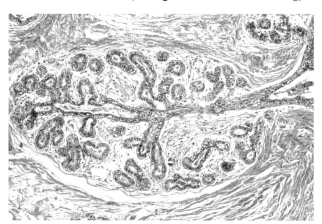

Fig. 1.5

Fig. 1.6

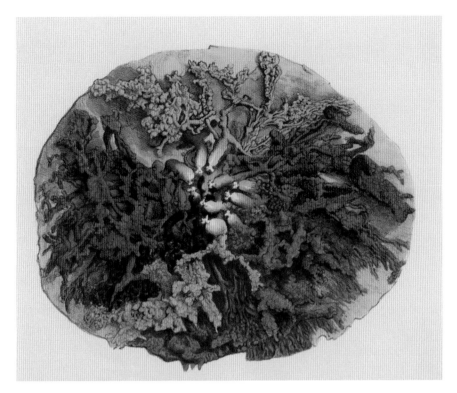

Fig. 1.7

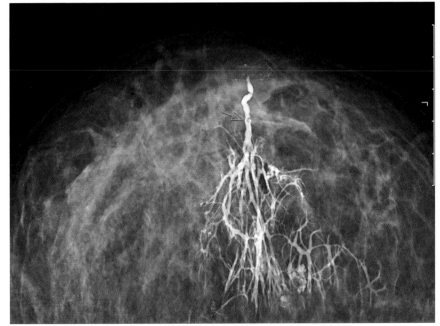

Fig. 1.8

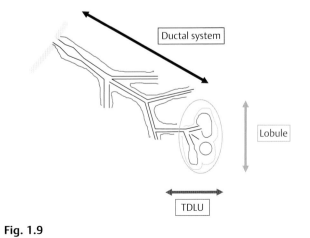

Fig. 1.9

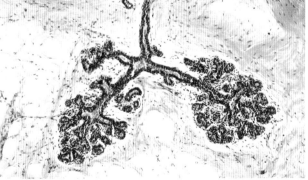

Fig. 1.10

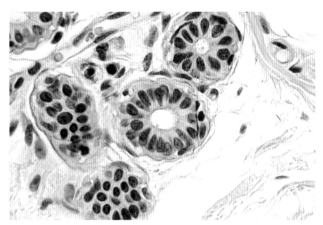

Fig. 1.11

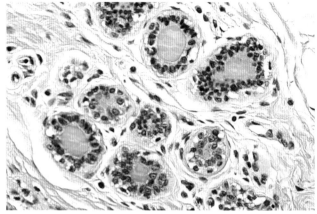

Fig. 1.12

The lobules comprise of many individual glands called acini and a hormone-sensitive special intralobular stroma. At the beginning of the menstrual cycle, the lobules are relatively small and contain only a minimal amount of secretion, if any, in the lumina of the acini (**Figs. 1.11** and **1.14**). During the secretory phase of the cycle, the acini produce eosinophilic secretions, and the intralobular stroma becomes edematous (**Fig. 1.12**). Around the time of menstruation, the myoepithelium becomes vacuolated and some epithelial and myoepithelial cells undergo apoptosis (**Fig. 1.13**).

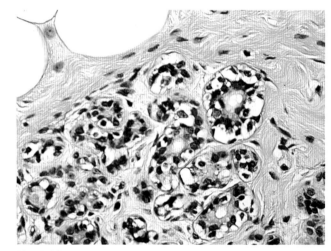

Fig. 1.13

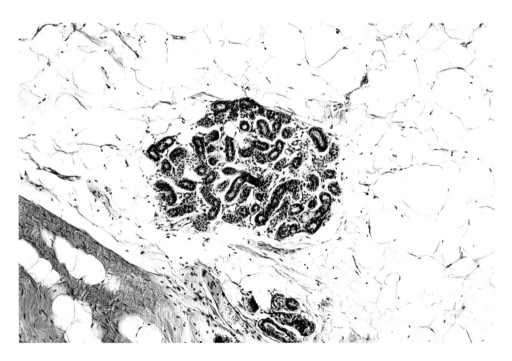

Fig. 1.14

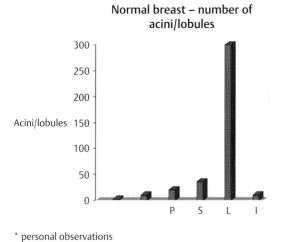

Normal breast – number of acini/lobules

* personal observations

Fig. 1.15

P—proliferative phase of the menstrual cycle
S—secretory phase of the menstrual cycle
L—lactation
I—involution

The most obvious changes are seen during the last trimester of pregnancy and during lactation when the TDLUs are enlarged, the number of acini per lobule increases greatly (**Fig. 1.15**), the cytoplasm in the epithelial cells becomes vacuolated, and rich secretions are produced in large quantities (**Fig. 1.16**).

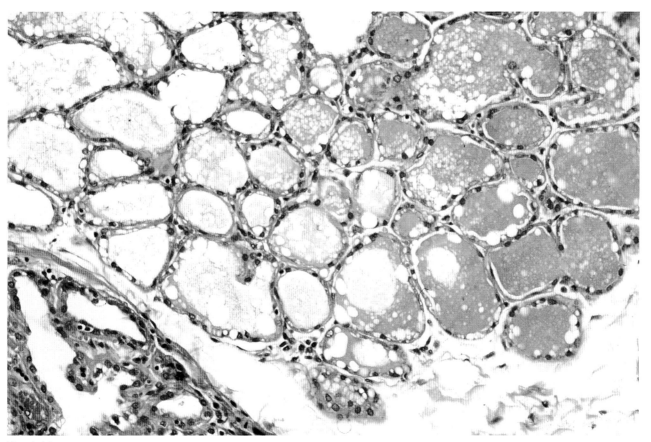

Fig. 1.16

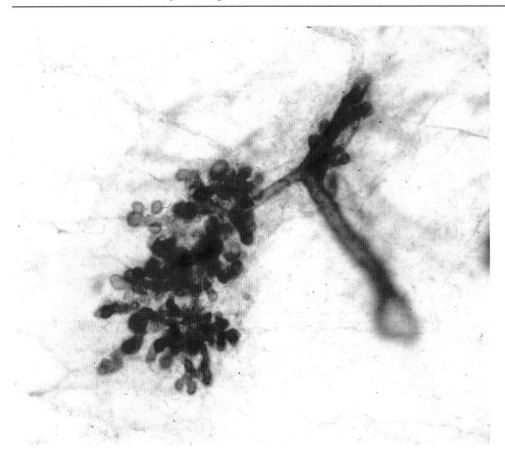

Fig. 1.17

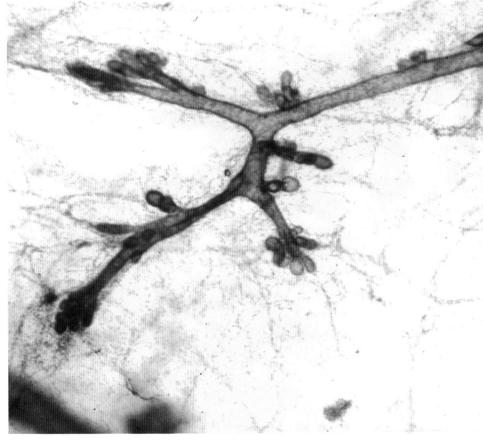

Fig. 1.18

Around the time of menopause, but often earlier, involution of the breast tissue occurs. Involution of the parenchyma results in a diminished number of acini/lobules, lobules, and ducts (compare **Fig. 1.17** showing a functioning lobule with **Fig. 1.18** showing an involuted lobule, thick-section images).

Fig. 1.19 shows a TDLU with normal mucin-rich intralobular stroma. Involution of the intralobular stroma is accompanied either by infiltration of fatty tissue (**Fig. 1.20**) or by fibrosis (**Fig. 1.21**). The same is true for the interlobular stroma.

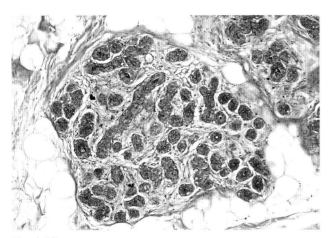

Fig. 1.19

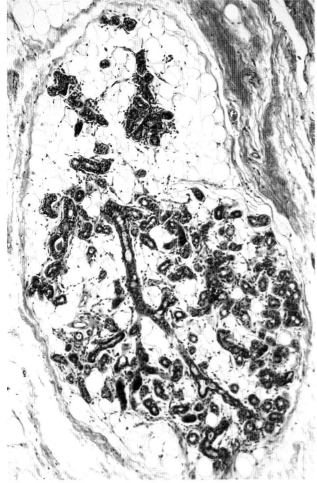

Fig. 1.20

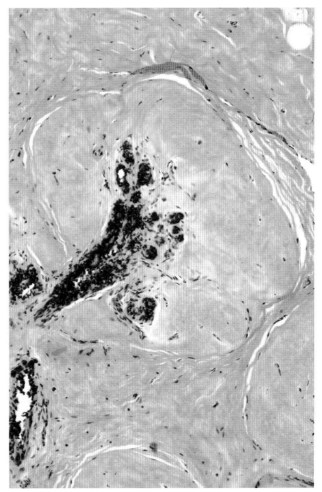

Fig. 1.21

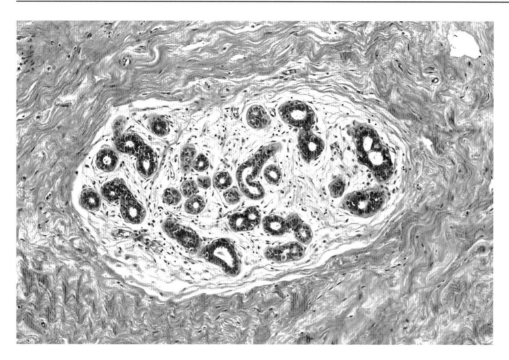

Fig. 1.22

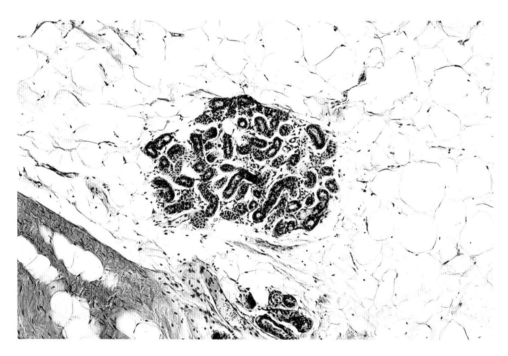

Fig. 1.23

The involution of the parenchyma and the interlobular and intralobular stroma is not necessarily a synchronized process. Functioning lobules can be seen in the presence of interlobular stroma that has undergone fibrous involution (Fig. 1.22) or has been replaced by fat (Fig. 1.23).

The intralobular and the interlobular stroma may undergo either fibrous or fatty involution in varying combinations (Figs. 1.24, 1.25, and 1.26).

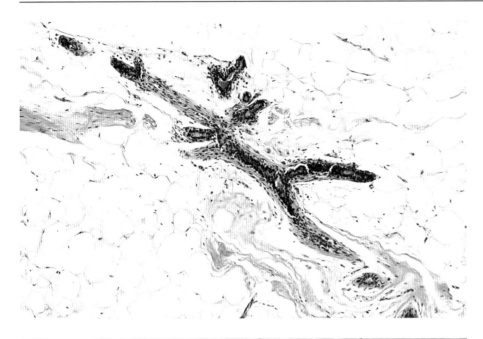

Fig. 1.24

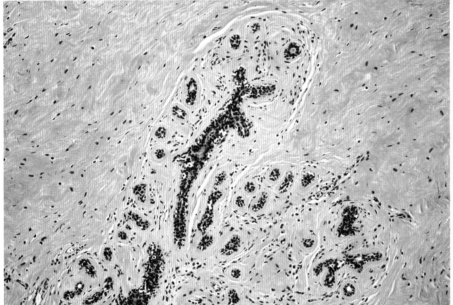

Fig. 1.25

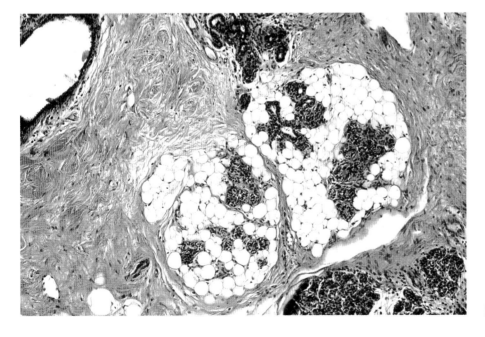

Fig. 1.26

The lobules may exhibit a different morphology from that described previously. This phenomenon is called aberration of normal development and involution (ANDI). The following are some examples of ANDI:

–   Apocrine metaplasia (**Fig. 1.28**) with large cells having granulated eosinophilic cytoplasm (as compared with normal epithelium, **Fig. 1.27**).

–   Clear-cell change (**Fig. 1.29**).

–   Eosinophilic change (**Fig. 1.30**), appearance of cells with eosinophilic cytoplasm among the cells of the usual type.

–   Lactational change (**Fig. 1.31**), milk-producing lobules in the breast of nonpregnant, nonlactating women.

–   Fibroadenomatoid change (**Fig. 1.32**) with the proliferation of the intralobular stroma and distortion of the acini.

–   Microcystic involution (**Fig. 1.33**, galactography image; **Fig. 1.34**, thick-section image; and **Fig. 1.35**) if involution of the lobules (diminished number of acini) is associated with dilatation of the acini.

A common type of ANDI is adenosis, which is described in detail in Chapter 6.

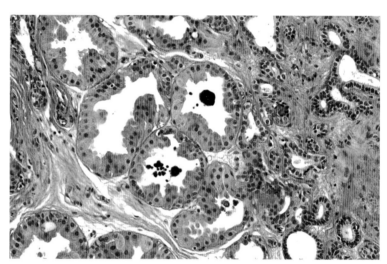

Fig. 1.28

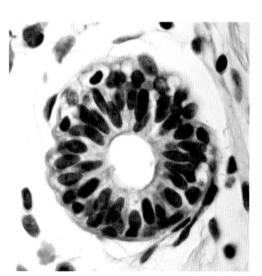

Fig. 1.27

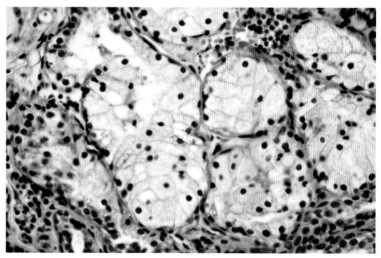

Fig. 1.29

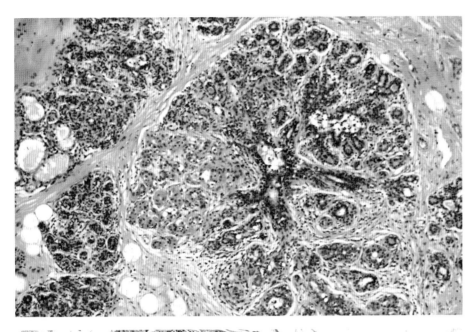

Fig. 1.30

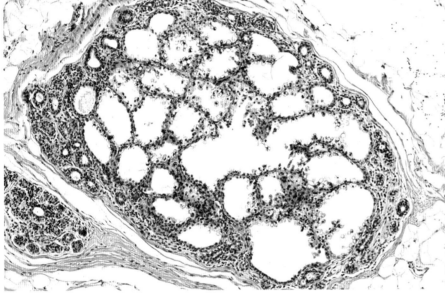

Fig. 1.31

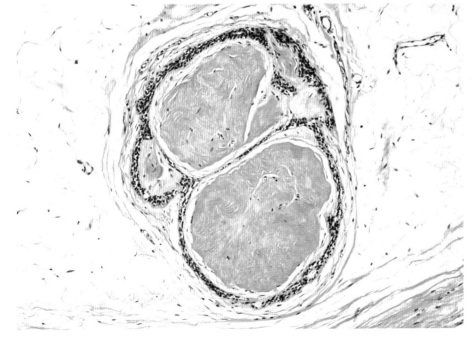

Fig. 1.32

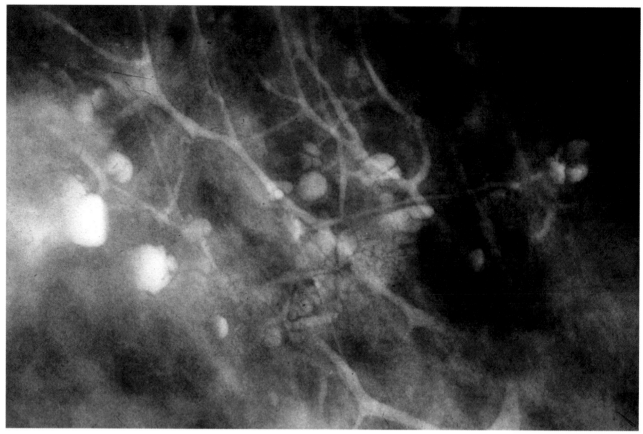

Fig. 1.33

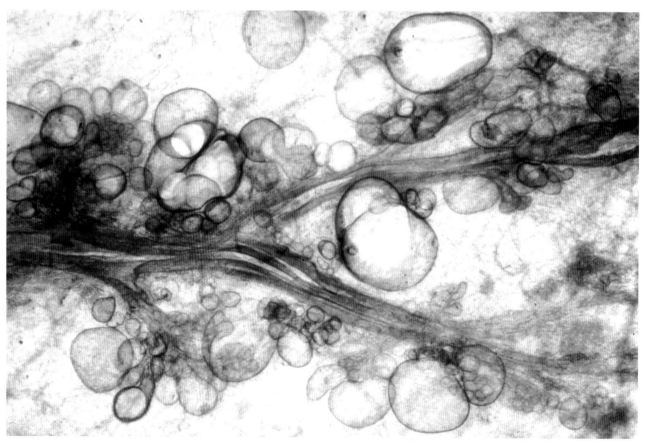

Fig. 1.34

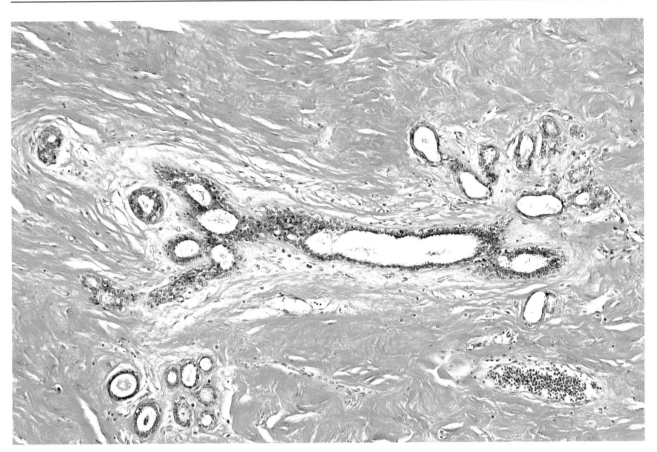

Fig. 1.35

Some ANDIs represent changes predominantly of the phenotype of the epithelial cells and may lead to accumulation of secretion in the lobule, which in turn may calcify. Other forms of ANDIs represent architectural changes within the lobules, leading to marked enlargement of the TDLUs. The microcalcifications associated with ANDIs may be seen on the mammograms and some of them may mimic malignant type calcifications causing differential diagnostic problems.

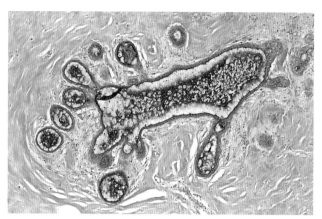

Fig. 1.36

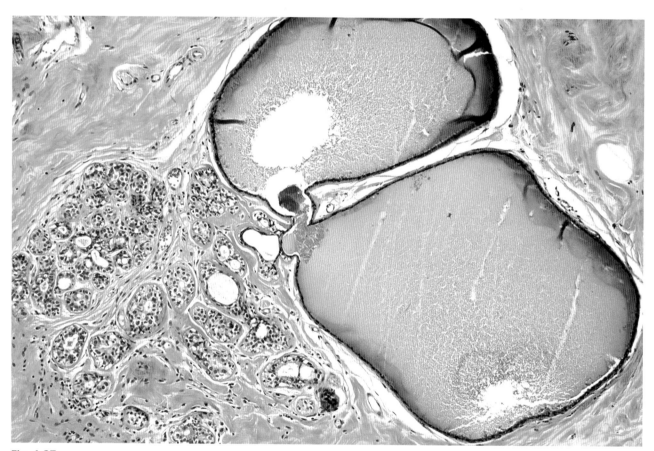

Fig. 1.37

The histologically "normal" breast tissue may show numerous aberrations, many of which cannot be detected by clinical or radiological examination. If these lesions are sufficiently large to be radiologically or clinically detected and especially if they are symptomatic, they are more appropriately referred to as fibrocystic change, which is still a variation of normal breast morphology.

The difference between ANDIs and fibrocystic change is more quantitative than qualitative. It is impossible to draw a sharp line between microcystic involution and cysts (**Figs. 1.36** and **1.37**) or between fibroadenomatoid change and fibroadenoma (**Figs. 1.38** and **1.39**).

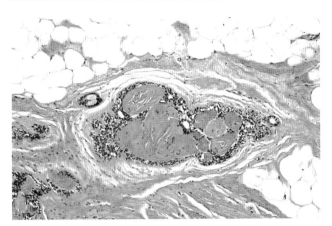

Fig. 1.38

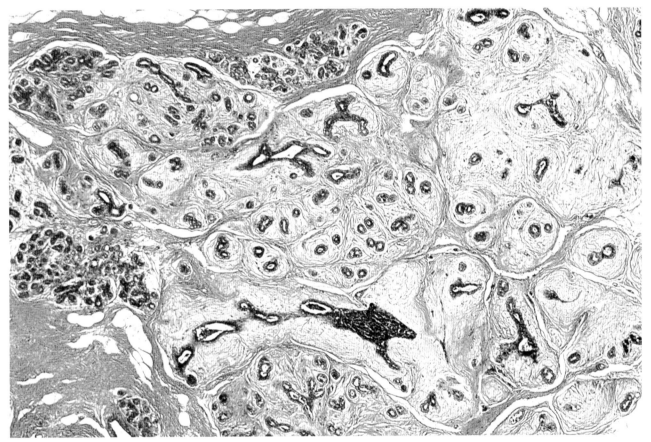

Fig. 1.39

The distinction between "normal" and "pathological" breast tissue depends on the method of examination. Histology is an extremely sensitive method and may detect many clinically and prognostically unimportant details, which are best characterized as variations and aberrations of the normal breast morphology.

The normal breast tissue may contain lobules typical of
both the proliferative and the secretory and menstrual
phases of the menstrual cycle, different combinations
of involutional changes, and different ANDIs, all
simultaneously. Consequently, normal breast tissue offers
the interested examiner a variable and fascinating picture
under the microscope [**Figs. 1.40, 1.41, 1.42, 1.43** (thick-
section image), and **1.44**].

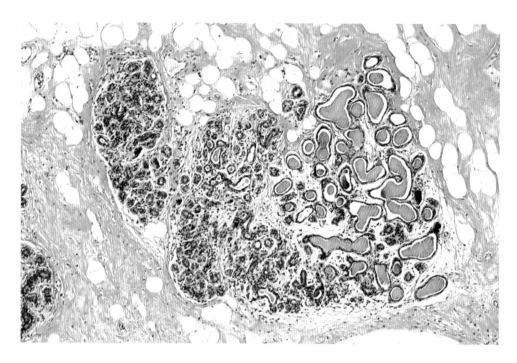

Fig. 1.40

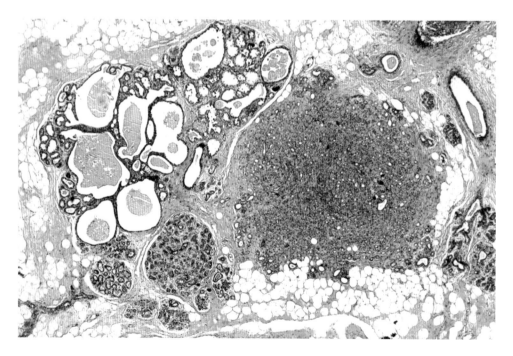

Fig. 1.41

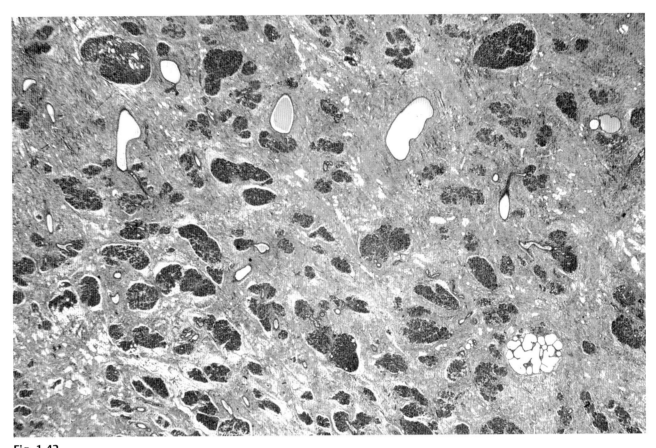

Fig. 1.42

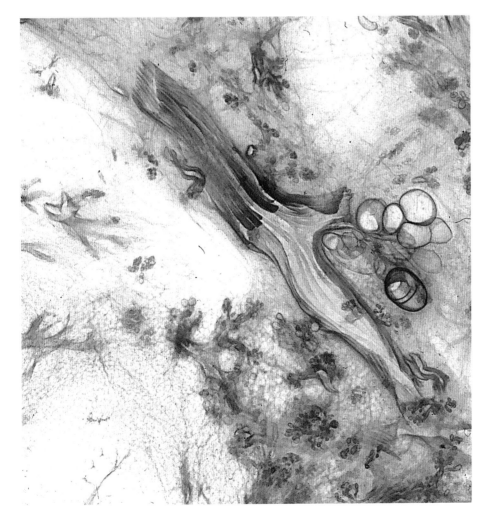

Fig. 1.43

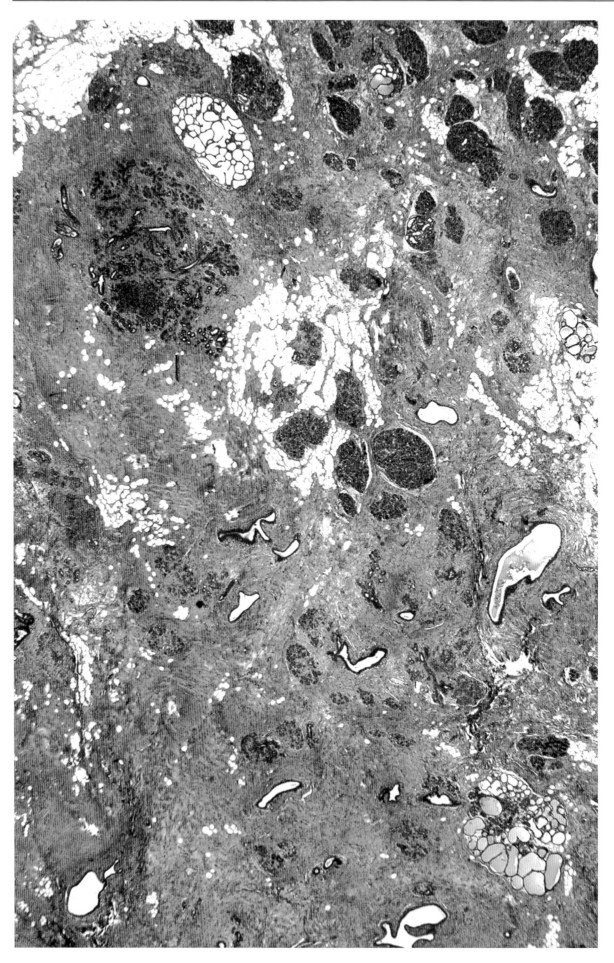

Fig. 1.44

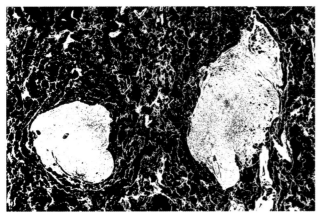

Fig. 1.45

The mammogram represents a black-and-white summation of the morphological details of the breast. The lobules can be seen as 1- to 2-mm nodular densities, which can cover a spectrum of histologic changes within the TDLU (**Figs. 1.45, 1.46,** and **1.47**). The ducts may be seen as branching linear densities on the mammogram, similar to vessels and fibrous strands (**Fig. 1.48**). The fibrous connective tissue appears as homogeneous, ground glass–like, structureless density, while the radiolucent fat outlines the radiopaque building blocks.

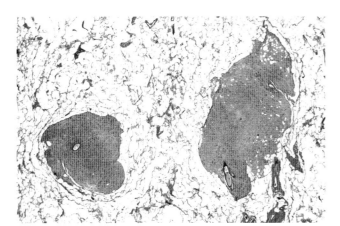

Fig. 1.46

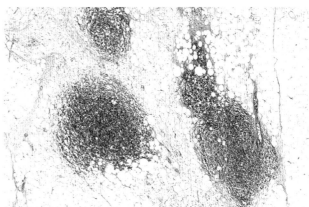

Fig. 1.47

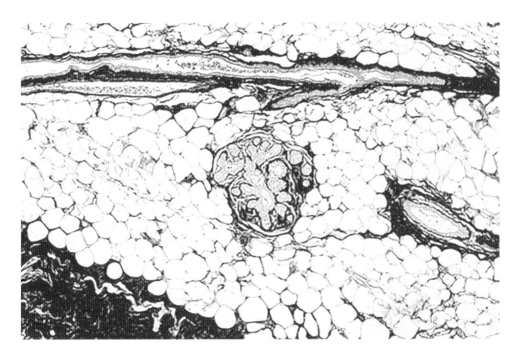

Fig. 1.48

The variable occurrences of these "building blocks" have been classified into five mammographic parenchymal patterns by Tabár and Dean. Gram et al correlated these patterns to epidemiologic risk factors. Tot et al correlated the patterns with the underlying histology image using large-format histology slides.

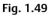

Mammographic parenchymal pattern I is characterized by Cooper ligaments and equal proportions of the basic building blocks (**Figs. 1.49, 1.50,** and **1.51**). The Cooper ligaments are composed of TDLUs, ducts, and fibrous connective tissue. One of the Cooper ligaments is marked in **Fig. 1.51**.

Fig. 1.49

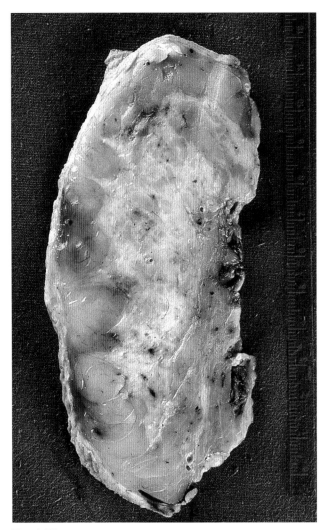

Fig. 1.50

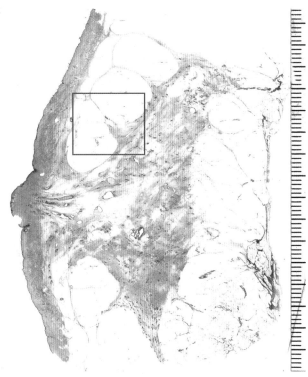

Fig. 1.51

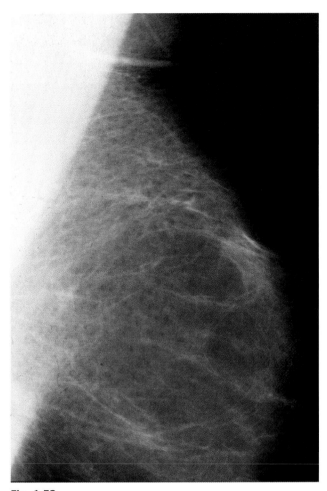

Fig. 1.52

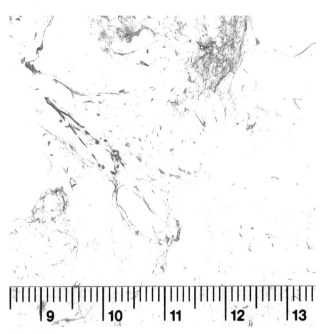

Fig. 1.53

Mammographic parenchymal pattern II represents fatty tissue outlined by fibrous strands with only a few remaining TDLUs and ducts (**Figs. 1.52** and **1.53**).

Pattern III is characterized by the presence of retroareolar prominent ducts with or without associated periductal fibrosis, extending to about one-fourth of the breast, which is otherwise replaced with fat (**Fig. 1.54**).

As the TDLUs and ducts involute over time, pattern I is transformed to pattern II or III. Hormone replacement therapy may convert pattern II or III back to pattern I.

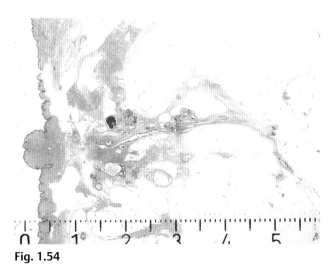

Fig. 1.54

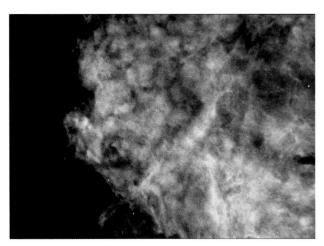

Fig. 1.55

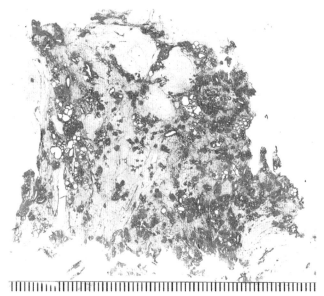

Fig. 1.56

Pattern IV is characterized by enlarged, 3 to 5 mm nodular densities and prominent ducts (**Figs. 1.55** and **1.56**). At histologic examination these nodular densities usually correspond to different ANDIs, but focal involution of the interlobular stroma with small islands of remaining fibrous tissue may present the same picture (**Fig. 1.46**).

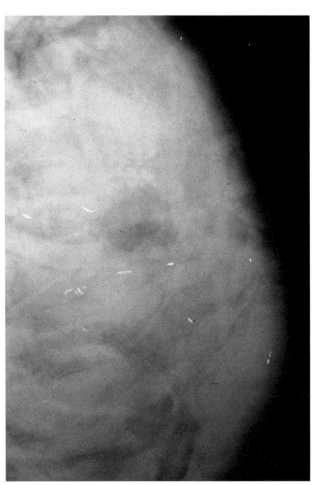

Fig. 1.57

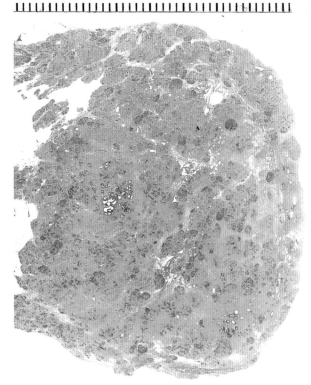

Fig. 1.58

Pattern V appears as a homogeneous, structureless radiopaque density covering most of the mammographic image corresponding to dense collagenous interlobular stroma, obscuring the TDLUs and ducts (**Figs. 1.57** and **1.58**). Patterns IV and V change little during and after menopause. Women having mammographic parenchymal patterns IV

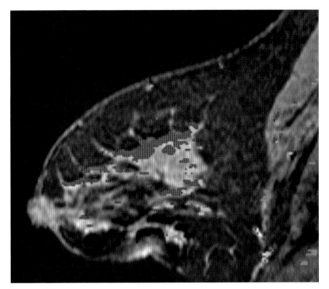

Fig. 1.59

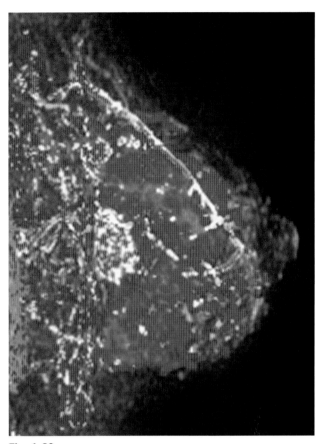

Fig. 1.60

and V have an approximately twofold risk of developing breast cancer compared with those of women having patterns I to III.

The Tabár classification is a qualitative classification system based on mammographic–histologic correlation. The widely used American College of Radiology Breast Imaging Reporting and Data System (BI-RADS)) quantifies the breast density into four quartiles according to the apparent relative proportion of radiopaque and radiolucent elements but does not relate the radiological patterns to anatomical variations of the breast tissue.

Magnetic resonance imaging (MRI) and modern ultrasonographic examinations are also able to demonstrate the parenchymal patterns with the basic building blocks of the breast tissue even in women with dense breasts (**Figs. 1.59** and **1.60**, MRI images). The Cooper ligaments are easily seen in **Fig. 1.59**; the background enhancement on **Fig. 1.60** is related to the high density of the breast tissue.

Conclusions

Comprehensive knowledge of the variations of normal breast morphology enables the pathologist to avoid overdiagnosing normal variations as pathological processes.

Clinical and radiological diagnoses assist the pathologist in the delineation of normal tissue from fibrocystic change.

The particular mammographic pattern of breast tissue is an important aid for the pathologist. Detection of pathological changes in breasts with patterns I, II, and III is relatively easy, but a more detailed histological analysis of macroscopically and radiologically normal breast tissue is necessary in patients with patterns IV and V.

Bibliography

1. Vogel PM, Georgiade NG, Fetter BF, Vogel FS, McCarty KS Jr. The correlation of histologic changes in the human breast with the menstrual cycle. Am J Pathol 1981;104(1):23–34
2. Longacre TA, Bartow SA. A correlative morphologic study of human breast and endometrium in the menstrual cycle. Am J Surg Pathol 1986;10(6):382–393
3. Hughes LE, Mansel RE, Webster DJ. Aberrations of normal development and involution (ANDI): a new perspective on pathogenesis and nomenclature of benign breast disorders. Lancet 1987;2(8571):1316–1319
4. Gram IT, Funkhouser E, Tabár L. The Tabár classification of mammographic parenchymal patterns. Eur J Radiol 1997;24(2):131–136
5. Tot T, Tabár L, Dean PB. The pressing need for better histologic-mammographic correlation of the many variations in normal breast anatomy. Virchows Arch 2000;437(4):338–344
6. Tabár L, Dean PB, Tot T. Teaching Atlas of Mammography. 3rd ed. Stuttgart/New York: Georg Thieme Verlag; 2001
7. American College of Radiology (ACR). Breast Imaging Reporting and Data System Atlas (BI-RADS® Atlas). Reston, VA: American College of Radiology; 2003
8. Going JJ, Moffat DF. Escaping from flatland: clinical and biological aspects of human mammary duct anatomy in three dimensions. J Pathol 2004;203(1):538–544
9. Tabár L, Tot T, Dean PB. Breast Cancer: The Art and Science of Early Detection with Mammography. Perception, Interpretation, Histopathologic Correlation. Stuttgart/New York: Georg Thieme Verlag; 2005
10. Hassiotou F, Geddes D. Anatomy of the human mammary gland: Current status of knowledge. Clin Anat 2013;26(1):29–48
11. Cooper AP. On the Anatomy of the Breast. Longmans; 1840, Plate VI

Chapter 2

General Morphology of Breast Lesions

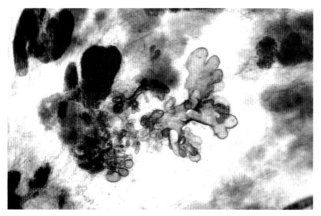

Fig. 2.1

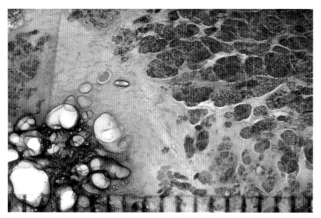

Fig. 2.2

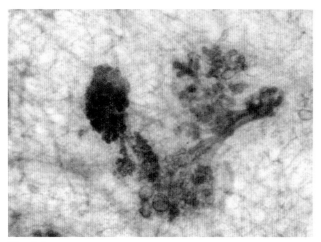

Fig. 2.3

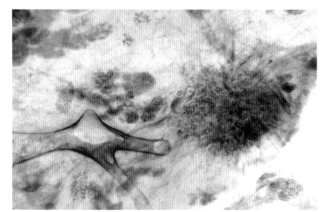

Fig. 2.4

General morphology describes subgross parameters assessable with both radiological and pathological methods. The results of these assessments are comparable to each other.

Most benign pathological processes in the breast originate in the terminal ductal–lobular units (TDLUs). The affected TDLUs become distended and distorted by the accumulation of fluid, mucin, calcium, or cells within the acini and/ or terminal ducts or by the accumulation of collagen, glycoproteins, and stromal or inflammatory cells in the intralobular stroma (**Fig. 2.1**, thick-section image). As described in Chapter 1, many benign lesions represent aberrations of normal development and involution (ANDIs) at the initial phase of their development and may become symptomatic as they enlarge. Benign lesions (such as papillomas) may also originate in the larger ducts.

Benign pathological processes tend to distend and distort the internal structures of the TDLU, but the contour usually remains spherical or oval, often with some lobulation (**Fig. 2.2**, thick-section image).

Malignant lesions may initially distend and distort the affected TDLUs, which can still retain their round or oval contour as long as the lesion is noninvasive (**Fig. 2.3**, thick-section image). Invasion destroys the preexisting structures at the site of development of the cancer in the majority of cases, and the contour becomes less circumscribed and more spiculated or starlike (stellate) (**Fig. 2.4**, thick-section image).

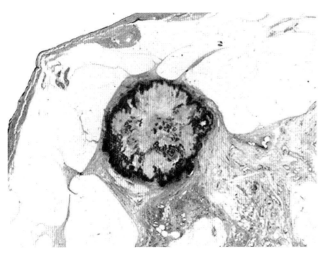

Fig. 2.5

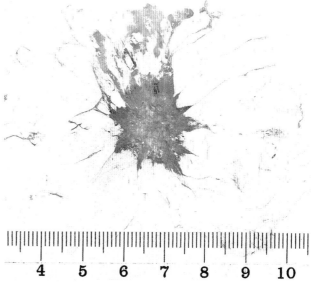

Fig. 2.6

As a result of distension or destruction of the preexisting normal structures, most invasive breast carcinomas are circumscribed round/oval masses (**Fig. 2.5**) or stellate masses (**Fig. 2.6**), and their size is relatively easy to measure. In neoplasia, the largest dimension of the largest invasive focus is considered to be the *tumor size*. This is a very important morphological prognostic parameter; patients with *early breast cancer* (defined as purely in situ carcinomas and those with the largest invasive focus < 15 mm) have excellent long-term outcome.

Asymmetrical invasion into the interlobular stroma, the appearance of additional invasive foci, and coalescence of these foci may cause the shape of the tumor to become increasingly complex. Some carcinomas are not circumscribed and grow diffusely forming a spider's web–like structure (**Fig. 2.7**). Similarly, cancers that originate in the larger ducts usually form a diffuse network (**Fig. 2.8**). Such tumors usually cause architectural distortion on the mammogram and seldom present as circumscribed mass lesions.

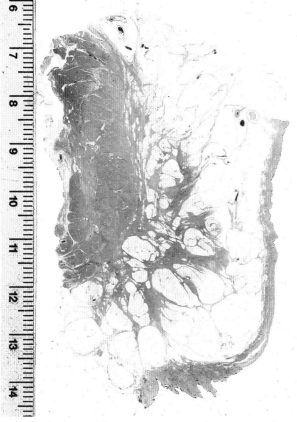

Fig. 2.7 (Reprinted from reference 4 with permission from the publisher.)

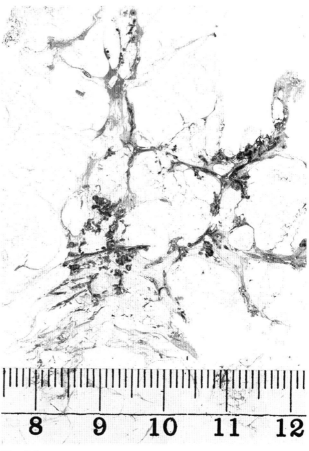

Fig. 2.8

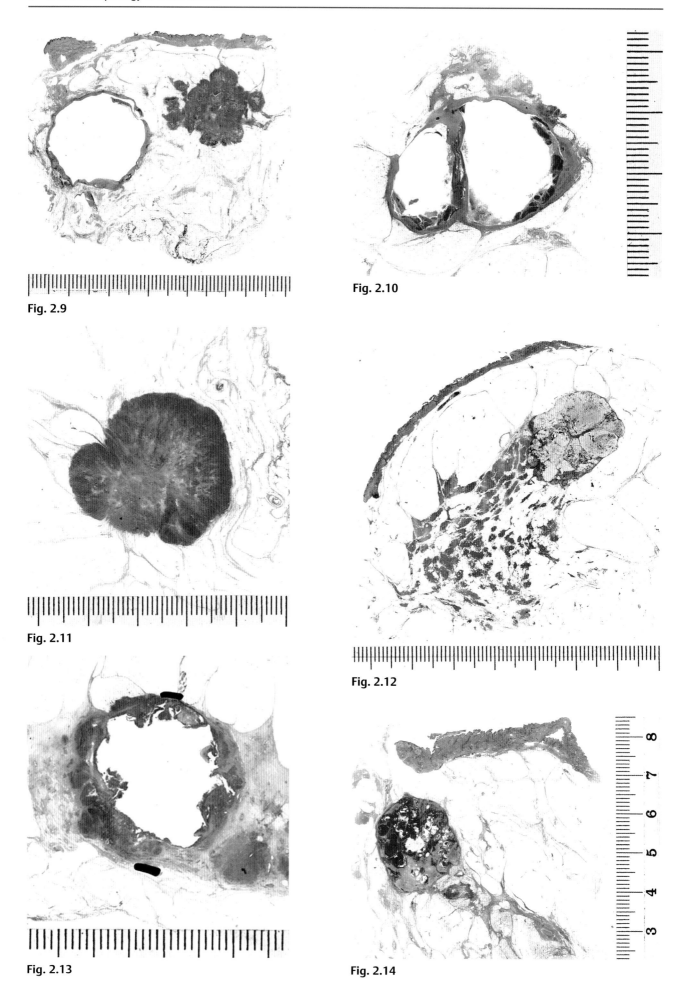

Fig. 2.9

Fig. 2.10

Fig. 2.11

Fig. 2.12

Fig. 2.13

Fig. 2.14

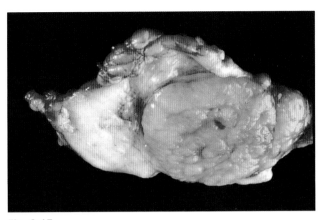

Fig. 2.15

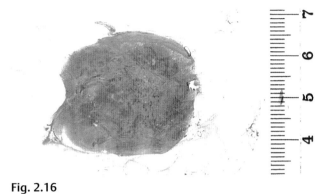

Fig. 2.16

The spherical/oval shape is not cancer specific and can be seen in benign processes including cysts (**Figs. 2.9** and **2.10**) and fibroadenomas; in malignant tumors such as medullary (**Fig. 2.9**), ductal (**Fig. 2.11**), and mucinous (**Fig. 2.12**) carcinomas; in tumors with cystic degeneration (**Fig. 2.13**); in metastases (**Fig. 2.14**); and in benign and malignant mesenchymal tumors (**Figs. 2.15** and **2.16**).

On the other hand, stellate lesions are nearly always malignant but may occasionally be radial scars or fibrous scars (**Fig. 2.17**, thick-section image).

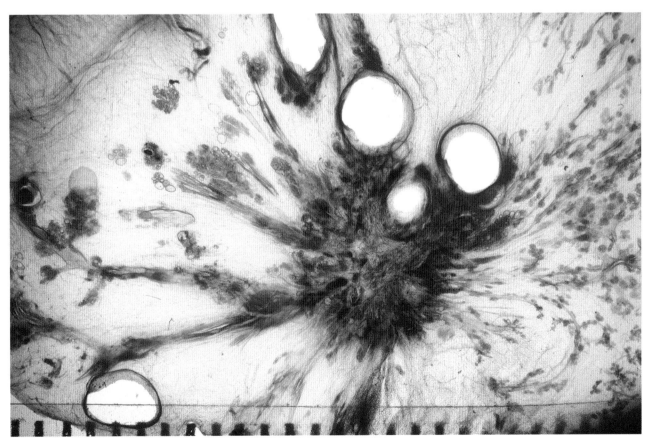

Fig. 2.17

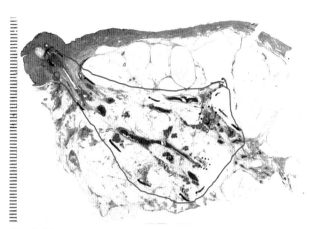

Fig. 2.18

Benign lesions may develop in any or all of the lobes of a breast, whereas breast cancer is a single-lobe disease. According to our sick lobe hypothesis, malignant lesions developing simultaneously or asynchronously originate in only one of the lobes. The lobar origin of breast carcinoma can be best appreciated during the in situ phase of tumor development (**Figs. 2.18** and **2.19**, same case), or in early invasive cancers (**Fig. 2.20**), whereas advanced invasive cancers often infiltrate the breast tissue beyond the structures of the sick lobe. Cancers of multilobar origin also exist but represent an exception rather than the rule. The sick lobe is presumed to have been damaged during embryonic development and is characterized by the presence of genetically altered stem cells, the so-called committed progenitor cells. Decades of accumulation of additional alterations are needed for complete malignant transformation of these cells, a process that may take place in any part of the sick lobe, both in the ducts and in the TDLUs. This transformation appears to be biologically timed and may involve one or more TDLUs, one or more segments, or most structures of the lobe, either synchronously or asynchronously.

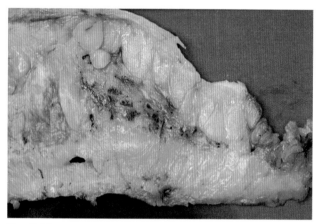

Fig. 2.19

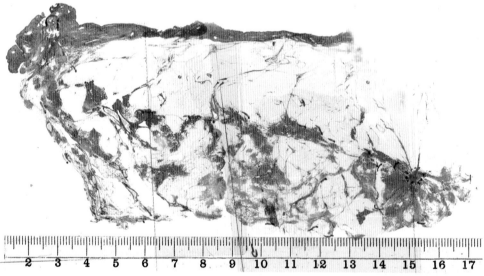

Fig. 2.20

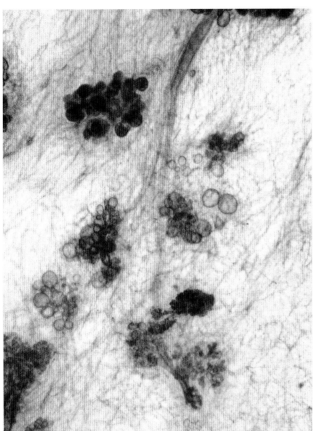

Fig. 2.21

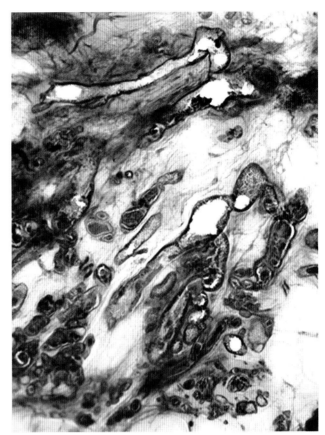

Fig. 2.22

In the majority of breast carcinoma cases the malignant transformation of the committed progenitor cells is restricted to one or more TDLUs of the sick lobe (**Fig. 2.21**, thick-section image), which indicates a good prognosis. On the other hand, in situ carcinoma that originates in the major ducts (with or without involvement of the associated TDLUs) (**Fig. 2.22**, thick-section image) is an important negative prognostic parameter. This prognostic impact of the in situ component is retained in the invasive phase of the tumor's natural history.

The malignant cells both replace the normal cells and take over their function. At the in situ phase of malignancy, the malignant cells are able to retain the basic normal ductal–lobular architecture of the breast parenchyma and the normal delineation of the parenchymal and stromal elements, although the involved TDLUs and ducts become enlarged and distorted. By accumulation of additional genetic alterations, the malignant cells may lose this ability, which leads to the tumor cells invading the stroma. A duct at the top of **Fig. 2.23** (E-cadherin staining) is an in situ structure. The central part of the image illustrates early invasion, and the structures in the distal end of the image are clearly invasive, no longer resembling normal ducts and lobules.

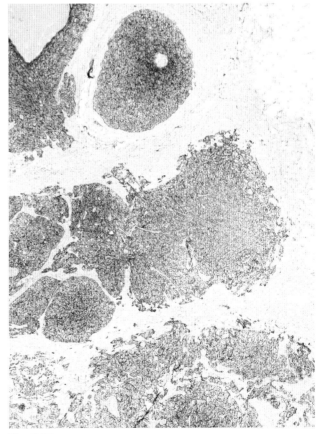

Fig. 2.23

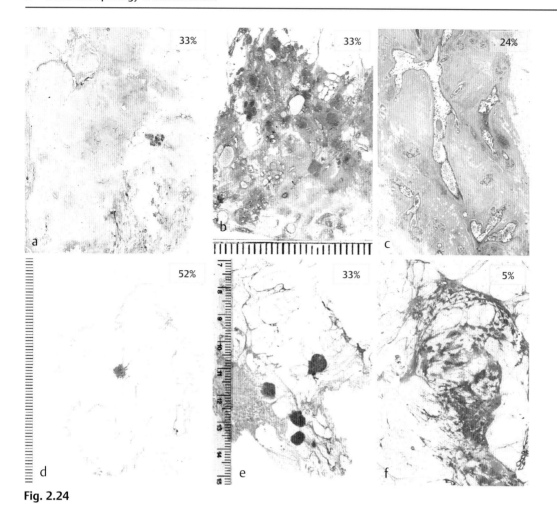

Fig. 2.24

Fig. 2.24 illustrates the possible spatial distribution of the in situ (**Fig. 2.24a–c**) and invasive (**Fig. 2.24d–f**) tumor components. The approximate case proportions are also provided from a large series documented on large-format histology slides. If the malignant process involves only a single TDLU or a few neighboring TDLUs and the associated subsegmental/segmental ducts a *unifocal in situ lesion* develops at the initial phase of the cancer's natural history (**Fig. 2.24a**). If the pathological process simultaneously involves more than one distant TDLU leaving uninvolved TDLUs in between, the in situ lesions are considered to be *multifocal* (**Fig. 2.24b**). If the process mainly involves the larger ducts (**Figs. 2.8** and **2.24c**), the lesion is considered to be *diffuse*.

If the invasion is restricted to a single focus within the breast, a *unifocal invasive* lesion develops (**Fig. 2.24d**). If the invasion happens synchronously at several distant points of the sick lobe leaving noninfiltrated tissue (normal breast tissue, benign lesions, or in situ cancer) in between the invasive foci, a *multifocal invasive* tumor component develops (**Fig. 2.24e**); the distance between the individual invasive foci is not of biological importance. Multifocality may also be a result of an intramammary metastatic process. The invasion of the stroma may also be *diffuse* if it happens simultaneously at many points of the sick lobe and if the interaction with the stroma is weak and insufficient to restrict the invasion to a well-delineated focus (**Fig. 2.24f**).

A considerable number of cases are detected in their in situ phase and there are also cases in which the in situ component is histologically undetectable. These cases were not included in the statistical values in **Fig. 2.24**. The vast majority, 75–80% of breast carcinoma comprises both an in situ and an invasive component. This fact clearly indicates the need for combining the individual distribution of the in situ lesions and invasive lesions into an aggregate (combined) growth pattern of the tumor (**Fig. 2.25**).

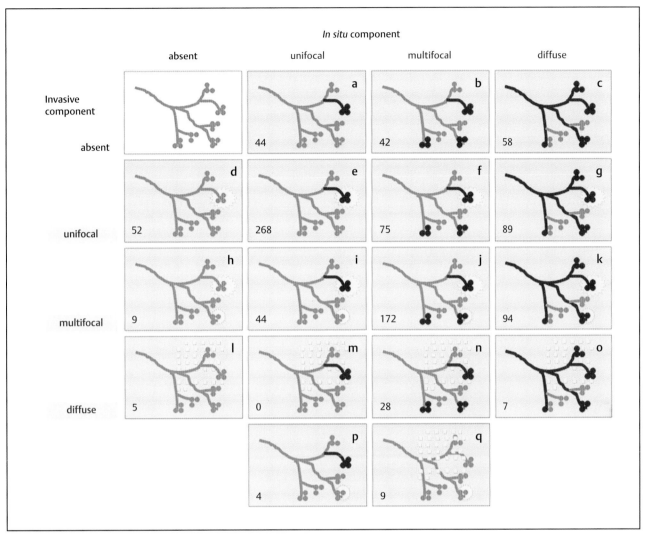

Fig. 2.25 Schematic illustration of the possible combined growth patterns in breast carcinomas. (a) Unifocal in situ component, no invasive component. (b) Multifocal in situ component, no invasive component. (c) Diffuse in situ component, no invasive component. (d) Unifocal invasive component, no in situ component. (e) Unifocal invasive component, unifocal in situ component within the area of the invasive focus, and unifocal combined pattern. (f) Unifocal invasive component, multifocal in situ component, and multifocal combined pattern. (g) Unifocal invasive component, diffuse in situ component, and diffuse combined pattern. (h) Multifocal invasive component, no in situ component. (i) Multifocal invasive component, unifocal in situ component in one of the invasive foci, and multifocal combined pattern. (j) Multifocal invasive component, multifocal in situ component, and multifocal combined pattern. (k) Multifocal invasive component, diffuse in situ component, and diffuse combined pattern. (l) Diffuse invasive component, no in situ component. (m) Diffuse invasive component, unifocal in situ component, and diffuse combined pattern. (n) Diffuse invasive component, multifocal in situ component, and diffuse combined pattern. (o) Diffuse invasive component, diffuse in situ component, and diffuse combined pattern. (p) Unifocal invasive component, unifocal in situ component outside the invasive focus, and multifocal combined pattern. (q) Drawing illustrating one of the possible mixed patterns with both diffusely growing and well-delineated invasive foci, with a diffuse combined pattern. The upper left image (unmarked) illustrates the sick lobe. Numbers in the lower left corner of the drawings indicate the number of cases in the series of 1,000 consecutive breast carcinomas belonging to that category. (Reprinted from reference 10, open access publication.)

Diffuse distribution of either the in situ or the invasive tumor components (or both) results in a *diffuse aggregate growth pattern*. Cases with no diffuse component but with a multifocal distribution of either the in situ or the invasive tumor components (or both) exhibit a *multifocal aggregate pattern*. The *unifocal lesions* are characterized by a single invasive focus with or without an in situ component within the invasive focus or in its immediate surroundings. **Fig. 2.25**

demonstrates the possible combinations of the distribution of the in situ and invasive lesions within the same tumor and the aggregate growth patterns. The number of cases belonging to each of the 17 categories in this series of 1,000 breast cancer cases documented on large-format histology slides and worked up with detailed radiological–pathological correlation are also specified.

As defined earlier in this chapter, *tumor size* is the largest dimension of the largest invasive focus. Another parameter, the *extent of the disease*, is also needed to properly characterize multifocal and diffuse breast carcinomas. This parameter represents the area or volume of the tissue that contains all the malignant structures within the breast. The size and the extent of breast carcinomas with unifocal aggregate pattern are similar or equal to each other. Diffuse breast carcinomas are better characterized by their extent because they do not form a well-delineated measurable tumor body. *Breast carcinomas of limited extent* (occupying a tissue volume < 40 mm in the largest dimension, **Fig. 2.26**), are appropriate candidates for breast-conserving surgery. Adequacy of breast conservation in more extensive tumors (**Fig. 2.27**) should be carefully judged preoperatively in every individual case. Carcinomas with an in situ component having lobar growth pattern (diffuse ductal carcinoma in situ) and invasive breast carcinomas of the diffuse type often represent extensive disease, limiting the success of breast-conserving surgery.

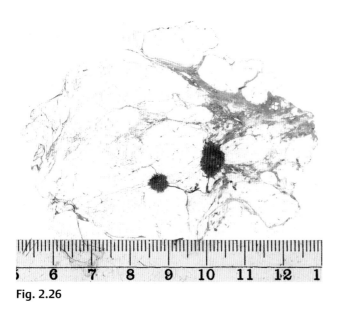

Fig. 2.26

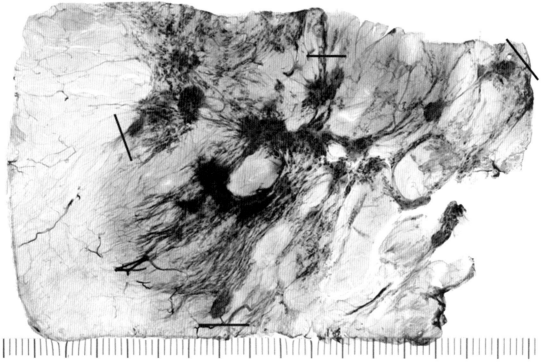

Fig. 2.27

Table 2.1 Early and more advanced breast carcinomas by aggregate growth patterns and disease extent, Dalarna County, Sweden, 2008–2012

	Unifocal	Multifocal		Diffuse		All
		Nonextensive	Extensive	Nonextensive	Extensive	
Carcinoma in situ	29% (60/208)	15% (32/208)	18% (37/208)	9% (19/208)	29% (60/208)	12% (208/1,654)
Early invasive cancer (< 15 mm)	40% (230/573)	12% (70/573)	22% (124/573)	6% (37/573)	20% (112/573)	35% (573/1,654)
Invasive cancer (≥ 15 mm)	37% (319/873)	10% (88/873)	25% (220/873)	5% (41/873)	23% (205/873)	53% (873/1,654)
All	37% (609/1,654)	11% (190/1,654)	23% (381/1,654)	6% (97/1,654)	23% (337/1,654)	100% (1,654/1,654)

As seen in **Table 2.1**, approximately half of the cases in a population with ongoing mammography screening belong to *early breast carcinomas* (purely in situ lesions and those with an invasive component < 15 mm in size). One-third of all cases have unifocal, one-third multifocal, and one-third diffuse aggregate growth patterns. Almost half of the cases are extensive (≥ 40 mm). These proportions are similar in both early and more advanced cases. These data are suggested reference values for quality assurance of radiological and pathological assessment of breast cancer subgross morphology.

The foci of a multifocal tumor are not necessarily identical to each other; they may differ in histological tumor type, grade, molecular phenotypes, and genetic characteristics. The resulting complex histological picture is an expression of *intertumoral heterogeneity* (**Fig. 2.28**, see also Chapter 9) seen in up to 30% of multifocal breast carcinomas. Different tumor cell clones may also occur within the same focus during tumor progression and dedifferentiation and lead to *intratumoral heterogeneity* (**Fig. 2.29**, see also case 1 in Chapter 10).

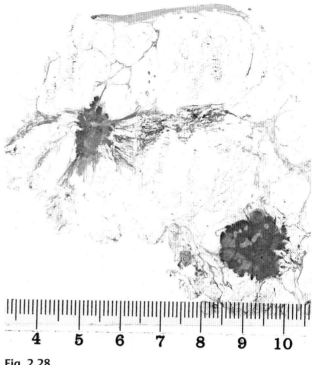

Fig. 2.28

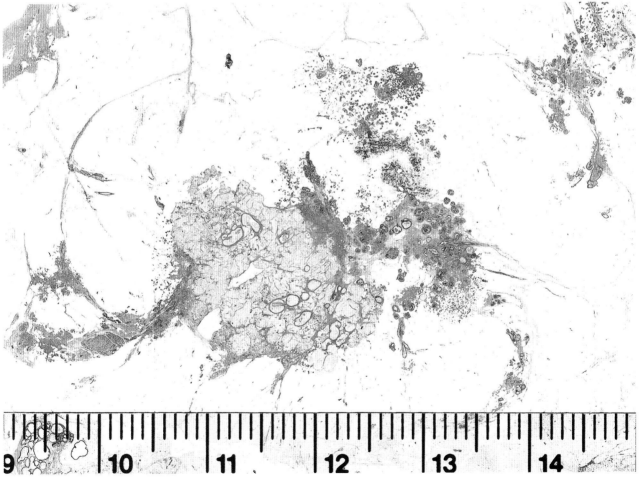

Fig. 2.29

The *location* of the lesions can be objectively determined by a combination of clinical, mammographic, ultrasonographic, and magnetic resonance imaging (MRI) parameters. To achieve uniform terminology, a horizontal and a vertical plane going through the nipple divide the breast into upper lateral, upper medial, lower medial, and lower lateral quadrants. In addition, a fifth area of the central, retroareolar cylinder is defined (**Fig. 2.30**). By applying different orthogonal projections when imaging the breast, the radiologist can measure the distance between the lesion and the nipple. Because the location of the lesion within the breast cannot be determined solely from a histological section, a system of marking the operative specimen is needed to provide orientation.

Mammography, ultrasonography, and MRI provide a good overview of the entire breast. The *size*, the *extent* (the involved area), the *distribution* (unifocal, multifocal, or diffuse), and the *location* of the lesions are usually well seen. Even when the lesions are not directly seen on the mammogram but are detected by indirect signs such as microcalcifications, the size, extent, distribution, and location of the lesions can still be well marked. The size, extent, and distribution of the lesions are well seen on the specimen radiograph postoperatively (**Figs. 2.31** and **2.32**).

Histological examination of the specimen is always necessary to further characterize the pathological process after the

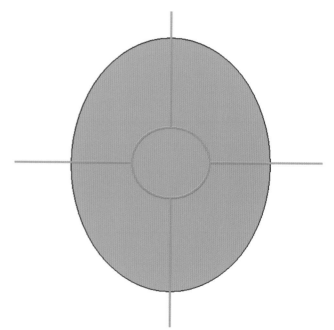

Fig. 2.30

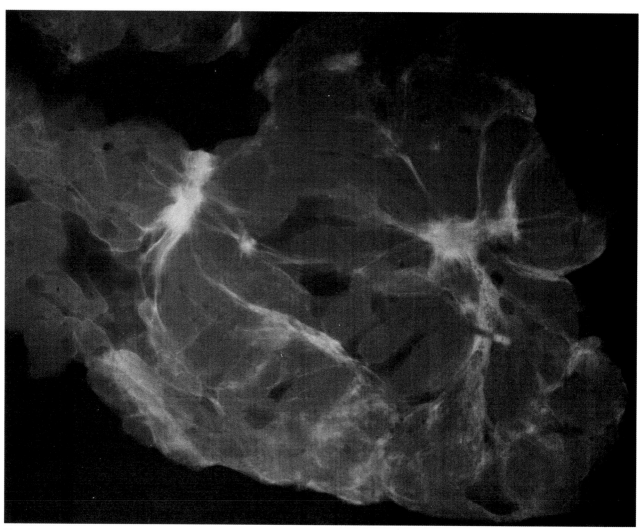

Fig. 2.31

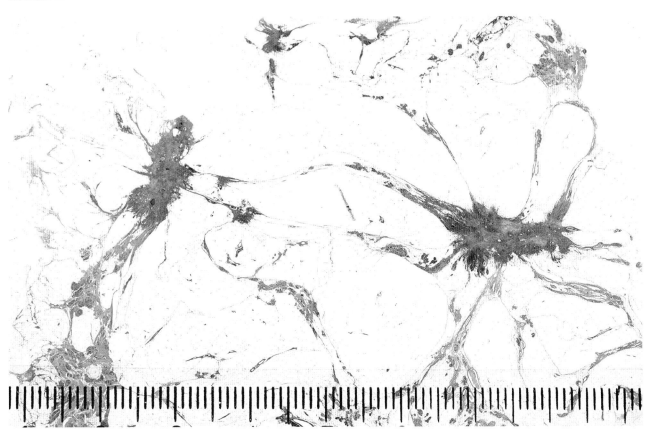

Fig. 2.32

tumor's size, extent, and distribution have already been indicated by the radiological methods. Histological examination should prove or rule out malignancy, confirm or modify the interpretation of the radiological findings, delineate the in situ and the invasive components, grade and type the tumors, reveal intratumoral and intertumoral heterogeneity if present, and provide further morphological prognostic and predictive parameters needed for therapy. Usually, and especially in cases of "indirect mammographic signs," the more sensitive method of histology reveals more details than the mammogram itself.

Conclusions

For a correct subgross characterization of a breast cancer case, the following parameters should be assessed: tumor size (defined as the largest dimension of the largest invasive focus), lesion distribution (unifocal, multifocal, or diffuse distribution of the invasive and in situ tumor components separately and in an aggregate pattern), disease extent (corresponding to the tissue volume containing all the malignant structures within the breast), intratumoral or intertumoral heterogeneity, and the location of the tumor(s) within the breast. These parameters can be assessed with radiological and histopathological methods, the most efficient being a combination of these methods in the form of detailed and systematic radiological–pathological correlation. Half of breast cancer cases are detected at an early stage (purely in situ carcinomas and invasive cancers < 15 mm) in a regularly screened population. Only one-third of breast carcinomas are unifocal (combined growth pattern), one-third consist of those with a unifocal invasive component and a nonunifocal in situ component, and in remaining one-third of cases multiple invasive foci are found.

Diffuse invasive carcinomas are rare, whereas a diffuse in situ component is present in a quarter of the cases. Half of the cases are extensive and occupy a tissue volume ≥ 40 mm in the largest dimension. The members of the breast team must be aware of the fact that the majority of both early and advanced breast carcinomas exhibit a complex subgross morphology.

Bibliography

1. Egan RL. Multicentric breast carcinomas: clinical-radiographic-pathologic whole organ studies and 10-year survival. Cancer 1982;49(6):1123–1130
2. Holland R, Veling SHJ, Mravunac M, Hendriks JH. Histologic multifocality of Tis, T1–2 breast carcinomas. Implications for clinical trials of breast-conserving surgery. Cancer 1985;56(5):979–990
3. Tot T. DCIS, cytokeratins, and the theory of the sick lobe. Virchows Arch 2005;447(1):1–8
4. Tot T. The subgross morphology of the normal and pathologically altered breast tissue. In: Suri J, Rangayyan R, eds. Recent Advances in Breast Imaging, Mammography, and Computer-Aided Diagnosis of Breast Cancer. Bellingham, WA: SPIE Press; 2006:1–49
5. Tot T. Clinical relevance of the distribution of the lesions in 500 consecutive breast cancer cases documented in large-format histologic sections. Cancer 2007;110(11):2551–2560
6. Tot T, Pekár G, Hofmeyer S, Sollie T, Gere M, Tarján M. The distribution of lesions in 1–14-mm invasive breast carcinomas and its relation to metastatic potential. Virchows Arch 2009;455(2):109–115
7. Lindquist D, Hellberg D, Tot T. Disease extent ≥4 cm is a prognostic marker of local recurrence in T1-2 breast cancer. Patholog Res Int 2011. doi: 10.4061/2011/860584
8. Tot T. The theory of the sick lobe. In: Tot T, ed. Breast Cancer: A Lobar Disease. New York, NY: Springer; 2011:1–17
9. Tabár LK, Dean PB, Tot T, et al. The implications of the imaging manifestations of multifocal and diffuse breast cancers. In: Tot T, ed. Breast Cancer: A Lobar Disease. New York, NY: Springer; 2011:87–152
10. Tot T. The role of large-format histopathology in assessing subgross morphological prognostic parameters: a single institution report of 1000 consecutive breast cancer cases. Int J Breast Cancer 2012. doi: 10.1155/2012/395415

Chapter 3

Hyperplastic Changes with and without Atypia

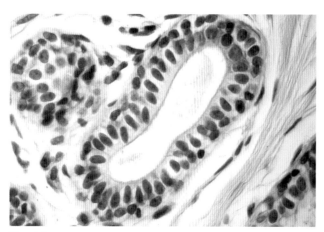

The normal ducts and lobules in the breast exhibit a single layer each of epithelial and myoepithelial cells (**Fig. 3.1**).

Fig. 3.1

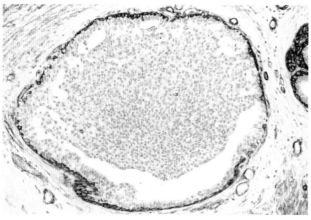

In epithelial hyperplasia, more than one layer of epithelial cells are present (**Fig. 3.2**).

Fig. 3.2

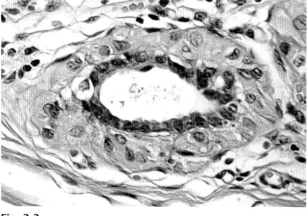

In myoepithelial hyperplasia, more than one layer of myoepithelial cells are seen (**Fig. 3.3**).

Fig. 3.3

Hyperplasia may be a focal or a diffuse phenomenon involving a portion of the terminal ductal-lobular unit (TDLU), the entire TDLU, or many TDLUs and ducts.

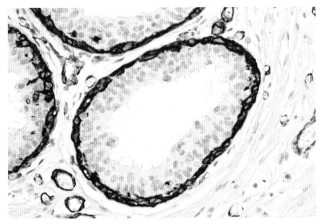

Fig. 3.4

Epithelial hyperplasia may result in the formation of only two to three layers of epithelial cells (**Fig. 3.4**), but often many layers of epithelial cells are present and form glandlike spaces or small papilloma-like structures ("florid" epithelial hyperplasia, **Fig. 3.5**).

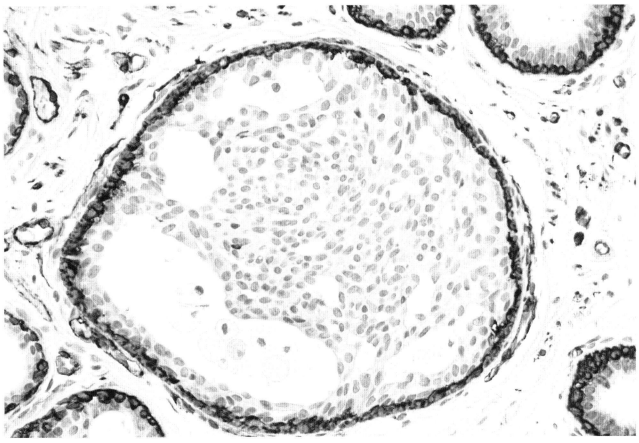

Fig. 3.5

Neoplasia may also result in several layers of epithelial cells within the ducts and acini. Hyperplasia and neoplasia can be differentiated on the basis of their cellular and architectural characteristics.

Cellular Characteristics

Hyperplasia is a benign proliferation of several cell clones resulting in a *polymorphous population of small cells* (**Fig. 3.6**).

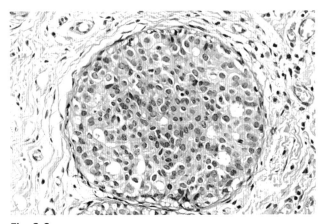

Fig. 3.6

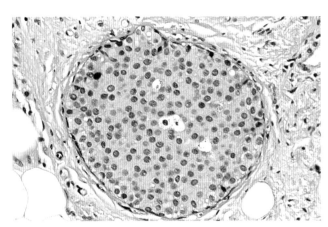

Fig. 3.7

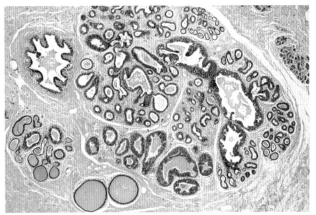

Fig. 3.8

Low-grade malignant epithelial cells appear as a monoclonal, *monomorphous population of small cells* (**Fig. 3.7**). These cells also give rise to several layers of cells within the ducts and lobules, resembling hyperplasia, and they may even appear within epithelial hyperplasia, partly taking over the structures. If only a portion of the TDLU is replaced by this monomorphous cell population, the lesion is called atypical ductal hyperplasia (ADH) (**Fig. 3.8**). If the entire TDLU is filled by the monomorphous small cells, the lesion is considered to be ductal carcinoma in situ (DCIS) grade I. ADH differs from DCIS grade I through extent and distribution, not through cellular features.

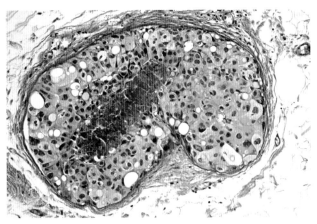

Fig. 3.9

High- and intermediate-grade in situ carcinomas consist of a *population of large and often polymorphous cells* (**Fig. 3.9**) and as such are easily distinguished from hyperplasia.

Architectural Features

The glandlike structures in hyperplasia are irregular, often slitlike, and of different sizes and shapes (**Fig. 3.10**). They become partly uniform and more "rigid" in ADH (**Fig. 3.11**), and regular and uniformly round or oval throughout the whole lesion in DCIS (**Fig. 3.12**).

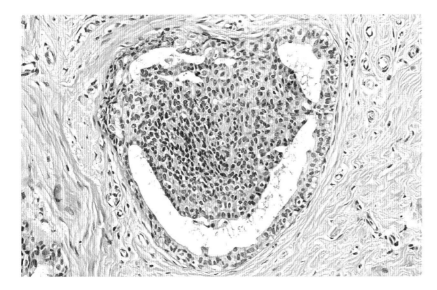

Fig. 3.10

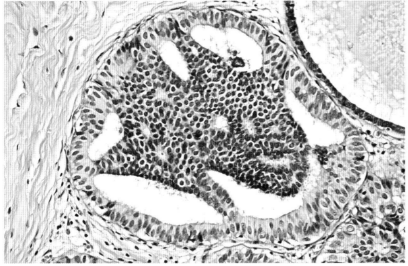

Fig. 3.11

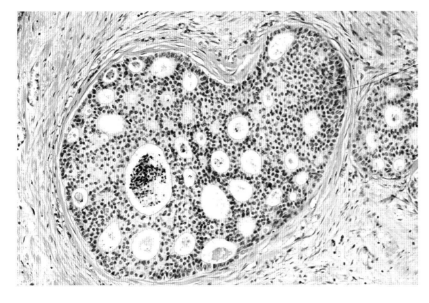

Fig. 3.12

An additional differential diagnostic feature is the polarity of the cells within the "bridges." In hyperplasia the cell nuclei are usually longitudinally oriented (**Fig. 3.13**), whereas in ADH and DCIS the cell nuclei are perpendicular relative to the axis of the bridges (**Fig. 3.14**).

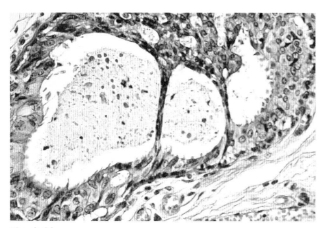

Fig. 3.13

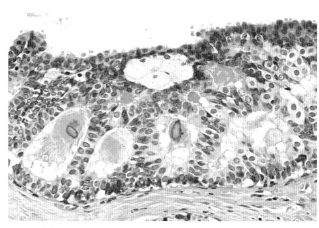

Fig. 3.14

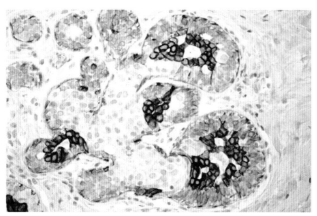

Fig. 3.15

As a polyclonal cell population, epithelial cells in hyperplasia often express antigens otherwise typical of myoepithelium (e.g., cytokeratin 5/6). These antigens are absent from the cells of ADH and most cases of DCIS. **Figs 3.15** and **3.16** show a TDLU partly filled with structures of epithelial hyperplasia (stained positively for cytokeratin 5/6) and partly with unstained malignant cells.

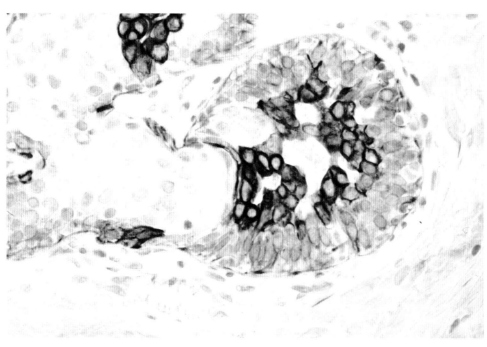

Fig. 3.16

Table 3.1 Summary of the features distinguishing usual ductal hyperplasia, atypical ductal hyperplasia, and ductal carcinoma in situ grade I

Hyperplasia	Polymorphous population of small cells Irregular glandlike spaces Longitudinally oriented nuclei in the bridges Myoepithelial antigens often expressed No restrictions on extent and distribution
Ductal carcinoma in situ (DCIS) grade I	Monomorphous population of small cells Regular, "rigid" glandlike structures Perpendicularly oriented nuclei in the bridges Myoepithelial antigens usually absent No restrictions on extent and distribution
Atypical ductal hyperplasia (ADH)	Features of DCIS grade I, with restrictions on extent and distribution Terminal ductal-lobular unit (TDLU) is only partly involved No more than two TDLUs are involved A single lesion is not larger than 2 mm

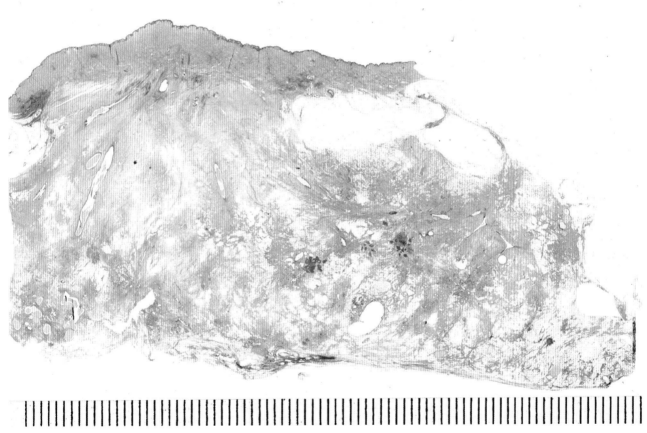

Fig. 3.17

Fig. 3.17 shows a borderline case between ADH and DCIS grade I: two TDLUs are involved, both are 2 mm in width.

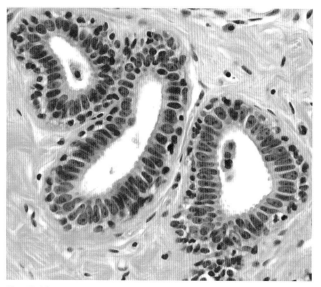

Fig. 3.18

Columnar cell change is a lesion characterized by one or several layers of tall cylindrical epithelial cells with cytoplasmic protrusions ("apical snouts") within the ducts and/or TDLUs. The single-layer variant is designated as columnar cell change (**Fig. 3.18**), the multilayered variant as columnar cell hyperplasia (**Fig. 3.19**). The cells may or may not exhibit cellular and nuclear atypia. The atypical variant of columnar cell change and columnar cell hyperplasia (**Fig. 3.20**) is also referred to as flat epithelial atypia because, in contrast to ADH and low grade ductal cancer in situ, micropapillary structures or glandlike spaces are not features of this lesion. Flat epithelial atypia is often associated with lobular neoplasia and low-grade invasive carcinomas.

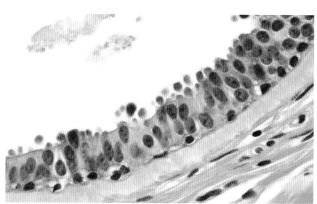

Fig. 3.20

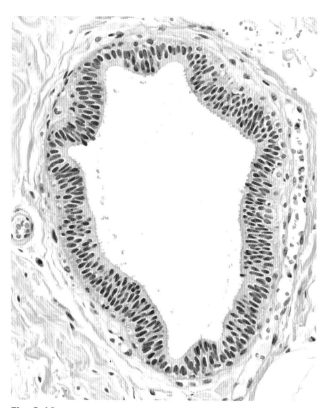

Fig. 3.19

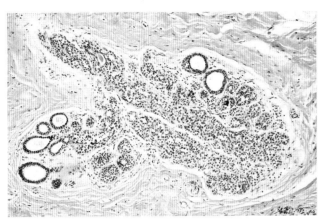

Fig. 3.21

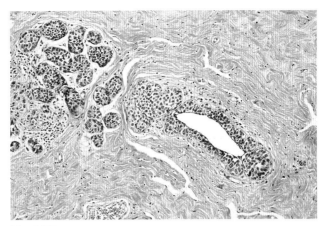

Fig. 3.22

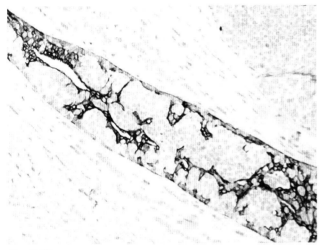

Fig. 3.23

The key feature of so-called lobular neoplasia is the appearance of a monomorphous population of small, loosely packed cells, which often contain a small intracytoplasmic vacuole that pushes the nucleus aside. These cells have the same appearance as the cells of invasive lobular carcinoma (see Chapter 5). Lobular neoplasia may originate in TDLUs as well as in the ducts. If only some acini are filled within the affected TDLUs while the others have an open lumen, the lesion is *atypical lobular hyperplasia (ALH)* (**Fig. 3.21**). If most of the acini within the TDLUs are filled with these cells, the lesion is *lobular carcinoma in situ (LCIS)* (**Fig. 3.22**). The typical pattern of involvement of the ducts by this process is formation of small intraepithelial nests of these cells in the wall of the ducts ("pagetoid spread") (**Fig. 3.23**, E-cadherin staining).

Hyperplasia, atypical hyperplasia, and neoplasia may originate in both the TDLUs and the ducts. Designating them as "ductal" or "lobular" is a more traditional way of discriminating two genetically and phenotypically different types of breast tumors: one consisting of cohesively packed cells building glandlike and papillary structures and the other consisting of loosely packed dispersed cells. All these lesions, hyperplasia, ADH, ALH, flat epithelial atypia, LCIS, and low-grade ductal carcinoma in situ are "borderline" proliferative lesions that represent either a marker of increased risk for subsequent development of invasive (usually low-grade) carcinomas or precursor lesions from which such invasive carcinomas develop. These lesions are often extensive, multifocal, or bilateral. Despite this fact, this low-grade pathway of cancer development is associated with a low risk of fatal outcome in the vast majority of cases.

Conclusions

Atypical ductal hyperplasia and flat epithelial atypia are "borderline" proliferative lesions very similar to ductal cancer in situ grade I and may represent the spectrum of the same disease. The same is true for atypical lobular hyperplasia and lobular carcinoma in situ. Although they are morphologically similar, they can be classified properly in most cases on the basis of established criteria.

Bibliography

1. Page DL, Dupont WD. Premalignant conditions and markers of elevated risk in the breast and their management. Surg Clin North Am 1990;70(4):831–851
2. Pinder SE, Ellis IO. Atypical ductal hyperplasia, ductal carcinoma in situ and in situ atypical apocrine proliferations of the breast. Curr Diagn Pathol 1996;3(4):235–242
3. Otterbach F, Bànkfalvi A, Bergner S, Decker T, Krech R, Boecker W. Cytokeratin 5/6 immunohistochemistry assists the differential diagnosis of atypical proliferations of the breast. Histopathology 2000;37(3):232–240
4. Schnitt SJ. The diagnosis and management of pre-invasive breast disease: flat epithelial atypia—classification, pathologic features and clinical significance. Breast Cancer *Res* 2003;5(5):263–268
5. Costarelli L, Campagna D, Mauri M, Fortunato L. Intraductal proliferative lesions of the breast-terminology and biology matter: premalignant lesions or preinvasive cancer? Int J Surg Oncol 2012;2012:501904

Chapter 4

Ductal Carcinoma In Situ

As mentioned in Chapter 2, the committed stem/progenitor cells and the cells of their progenies in this phase of development of the cancer are still able to maintain the normal ductal–lobular architecture of the parenchyma during the constant renewal of the breast tissue. The dimorphic, epithelial–myoepithelial differentiation of these cells is also maintained, as well as the delineation of the parenchyma and stroma with a continuous basement membrane.

> Carcinoma in situ is a malignant tumor growing in spaces surrounded by an intact basement membrane.

These spaces are either preformed, preexisting ducts or lobules, or newly formed acini, lobules, or ducts (**Fig. 4.1**).

The diagnostic criteria for carcinoma in situ are as follows:

– Intact basement membrane (**Figs. 4.2** and **4.3**, digital inversion of the image in **Fig. 4.2**)

– Malignant cells not invading through the basement membrane

Malignancy of the tumor cells can be illustrated immunohistochemically; for example, by staining on oncogene c-erbB-2 (HER2) in many cases (**Fig. 4.5**).

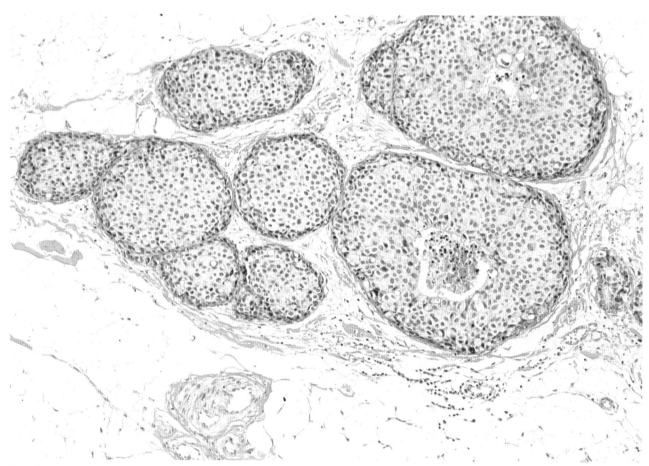

Fig. 4.1

The criterion of an intact basement membrane (**Figs. 4.2** and **4.3**) is more accurate for determining the non-invasive character of breast carcinoma because the myoepithelial cell layer may be discontinuous or focally absent (**Fig. 4.4**, smooth muscle actin stain).

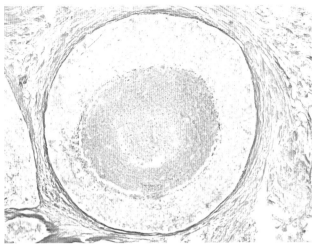

Fig. 4.2

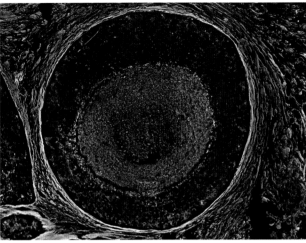

Fig. 4.3

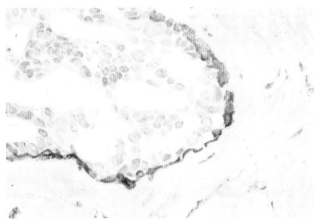

Fig. 4.4

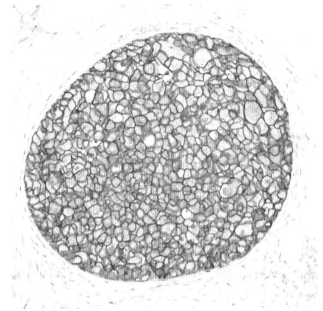

Fig. 4.5

Cancer in situ may develop in any part of the sick breast lobe, more often in terminal ductal-lobular units (TDLUs) than in larger ducts. The widely used terms *ductal carcinoma in situ (DCIS)* and *lobular carcinoma in situ (LCIS)* initially proposed to designate the site of origin of the process are not valid in this meaning. The word *ductal* indicates a tissue differentiation other than *lobular. Ductal differentiation* means that the tumor cells are larger and more cohesive with a tendency to form glandlike or papillary structures. LCIS on the other hand contains smaller cells, often with a cytoplasmic vacuole; these cells are less cohesive and never form glandlike or papillary structures (see also Chapter 3). There are substantial differences in genetic and phenotypic characteristics of the tumors showing ductal and lobular differentiation; for example, most ductal carcinomas express E-cadherin, in contrast to lobular ones. These characteristics allow the pathologist to delineate the two basic types of carcinoma in situ, DCIS and LCIS, in the vast majority of cases. However, DCIS and LCIS often coexist, and rare hybrid cases showing both ductal and lobular differentiation also occur (**Fig. 4.6**, E-cadherin stain). DCIS itself, most often detected by mammographic examination, is a heterogeneous disease. The numerous subtypes have specific radiological appearances matching the differences in the underlying histology. The histologic diagnosis needs to be further stratified by grading and subtyping.

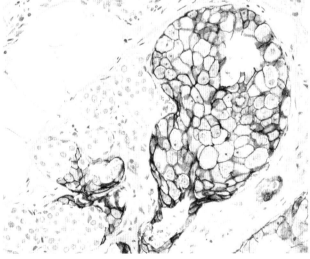

Fig. 4.6

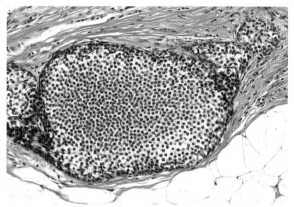

Fig. 4.7

When grading DCIS, the most important histopathologic prognostic factor is the *nuclear grade*, as follows:

– *Low nuclear grade*: monomorphous, small nuclei, no or very few regular mitoses, no or few apoptotic bodies (**Fig. 4.7**). The nuclei are usually diploid and estrogen-receptor positive.

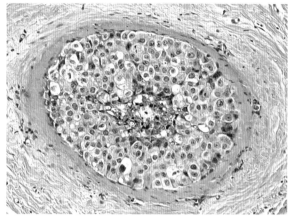

Fig. 4.8

– *High nuclear grade*: polymorphous, large nuclei with high mitotic rate and many apoptotic bodies (**Fig. 4.8**). Irregular mitoses can be present. The nuclei are usually aneuploid and estrogen-receptor negative.

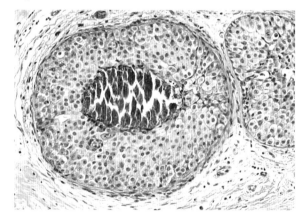

Fig. 4.9

– *Intermediate nuclear grade*: somewhat enlarged and somewhat polymorphous nuclei with few mitoses and few apoptotic bodies (**Fig. 4.9**).

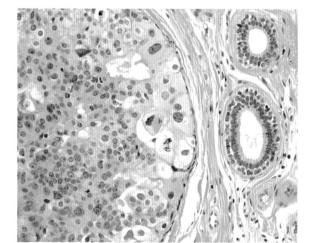

Fig. 4.10

The nuclear grade may vary considerably in the same DCIS (**Fig. 4.10**). In these cases, the use of the highest nuclear grade is recommended.

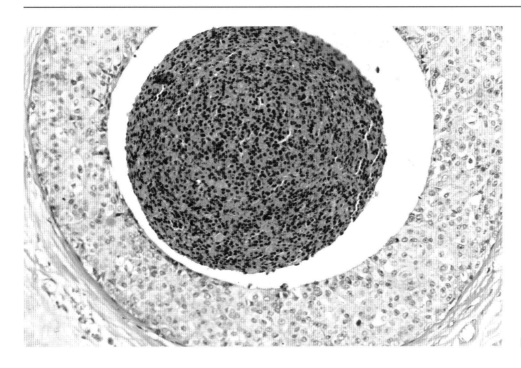

Fig. 4.11

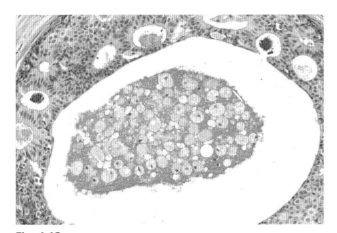

Fig. 4.12

The second most important histopathologic prognostic factor in grading DCIS is the presence or absence of *central necrosis* in the lumen of the ducts and acini. This necrosis is the result of cell death, as indicated by the presence of apoptotic nuclear fragments in the necrotic debris (**Fig. 4.11**). Secretion in the lumen of the ducts with DCIS, which often contain degenerated cells (**Fig. 4.12**), must be recognized as not representing necrosis.

A simple practical grading system of DCIS is recommended, as follows:

– DCIS grade I: low nuclear grade without central necrosis

– DCIS grade II: low nuclear grade with central necrosis, or intermediate nuclear grade (with or without central necrosis)

– DCIS grade III: high nuclear grade (with or without central necrosis)

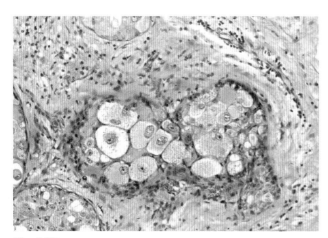

Fig. 4.13

The tumor cells of DCIS may express phenotypic variations enabling the recognition of DCIS subtypes, as follows:

– Apocrine DCIS (**Fig. 4.13**)

– Endocrine DCIS (**Fig. 4.14**)

– Clear-cell DCIS (**Fig. 4.15**)

– Signet-ring cell DCIS (**Fig. 4.16**)

This subtyping, though morphologically simple and straightforward, has only minimal clinical value.

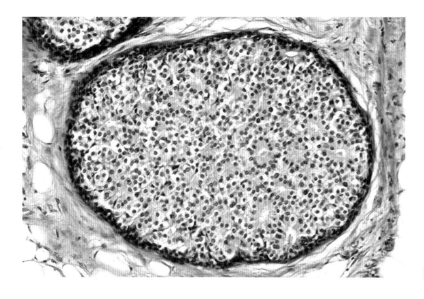

Fig. 4.14

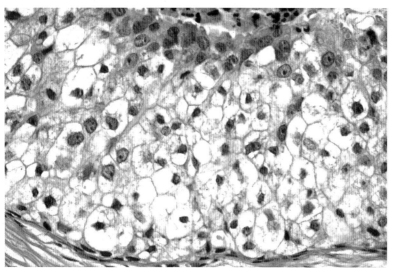

Fig. 4.15

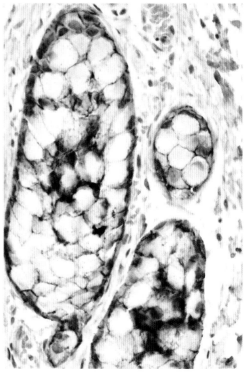

Fig. 4.16

The growth pattern of DCIS is important to the histologist for the differential diagnosis of DCIS, benign hyperplasia, atypical ductal hyperplasia, and LCIS. The patterns are as follows:

- Micropapillary DCIS (**Fig. 4.17**)
- Cribriform DCIS (**Fig. 4.18**)
- Solid DCIS (**Fig. 4.19**)
- Clinging DCIS (**Fig. 4.20**)

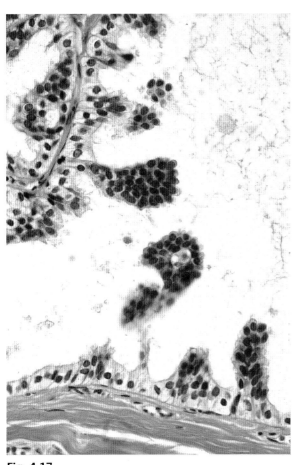

Fig. 4.17

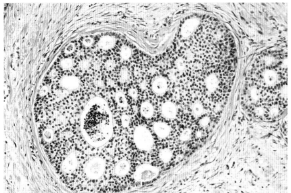

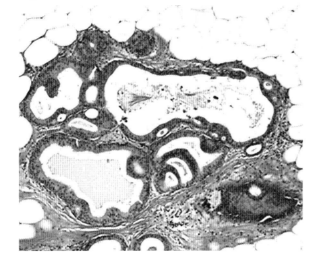

Fig. 4.18

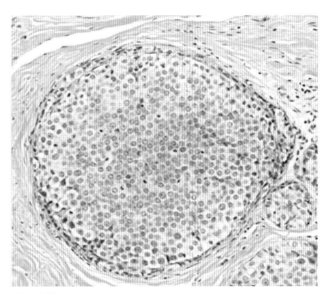

Fig. 4.19

Any histologic growth pattern can be associated with low, intermediate, and high nuclear grade and may or may not show central necrosis. The growth pattern, the histologic malignancy grade, the presence or absence of necrosis or fluid production all influence the mammographic appearance of cancer in situ as well as the clinical picture. Micropapillary DCIS is often more extensive than in situ tumors showing other growth patterns.

Fig. 4.20

The central necrotic material often becomes dystrophically calcified, forming large, irregular, elongated, or triangular and frequently quite extensive *amorphous microcalcifications* (**Figs. 4.21** and **4.22**), which can be readily visualized on the mammogram.

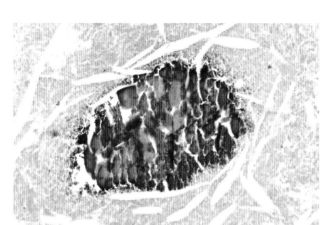

Fig. 4.21

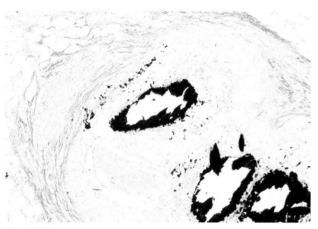

Fig. 4.22

The secretions in the lumen of DCIS grade I may calcify and form *psammoma bodies* (**Fig. 4.25**), which are small and laminated and are detectable on the mammogram as clustered *powdery microcalcifications* only when numerous (**Fig. 4.26**).

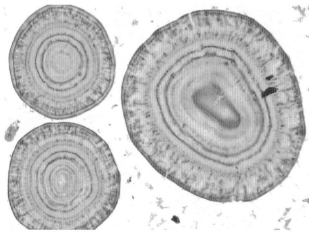

Fig. 4.25

The amorphous calcifications of DCIS tend to gradually fill the ducts and appear as long, branching calcifications on the mammogram, the so-called casting type calcifications (**Fig. 4.23**). If the cancer in situ fills a dilated lobule, the calcifications may appear as triangular or "broken-needle type" ("crushed stone–like") (**Fig. 4.24**), often in clusters.

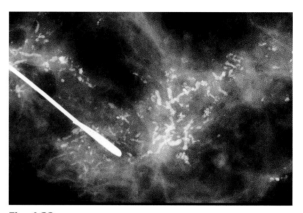

Fig. 4.23

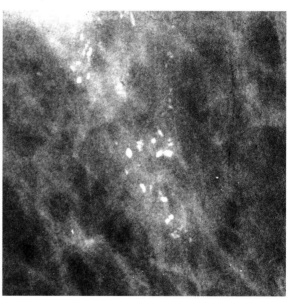

Fig. 4.24

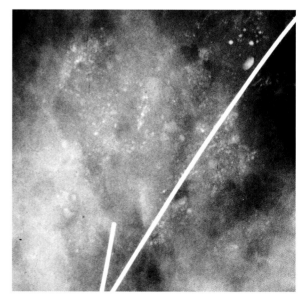

Fig. 4.26

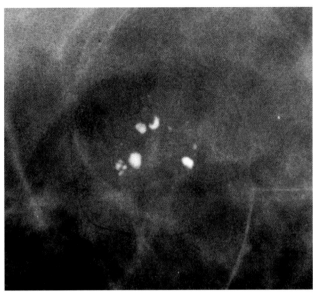

Fig. 4.27

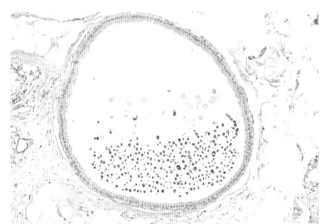

Fig. 4.28

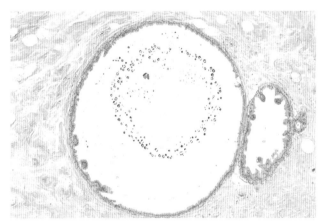

Fig. 4.29

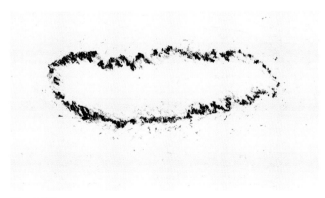

Fig. 4.30

Microcalcifications appear in many benign conditions in the breast. In fibrocystic change, the microcalcifications can be teacup-like (**Figs. 4.27, 4.28,** and **4.29**), weddellites (calcium oxalate crystals) or "skipping stone–like" calcifications. Whereas the casting type of microcalcifications is almost specific for DCIS, clusters of the broken-needle type of calcifications may appear in fibroadenomas, fibrocystic change, or papillomas. Powdery microcalcifications are often seen in sclerosing adenosis. Calcified arteries typically appear as double linear calcifications (**Fig. 4.30**).

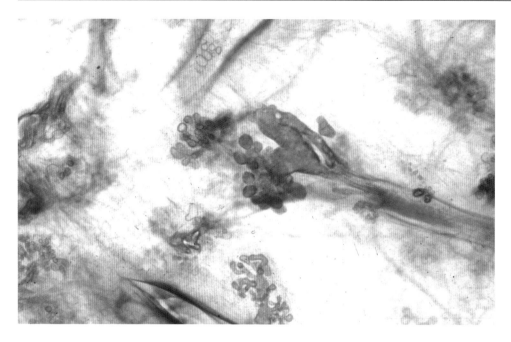

Fig. 4.31

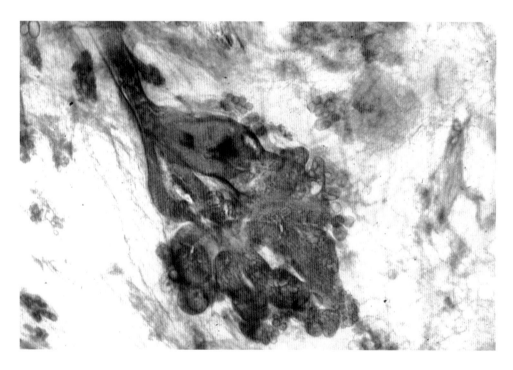

Fig. 4.32

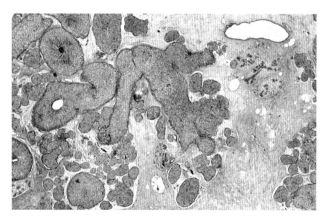

In less aggressive cases of ductal carcinoma in situ, the tumor does not leave the TDLU but causes dilatation and distortion of the affected TDLU (**Figs. 4.31** and **4.32**, thick-section images). In more aggressive cases of DCIS, the tumor engages the neighboring ducts and TDLUs, growing into the lumen of the normal acini (the so-called cancerization of the lobules) (**Fig. 4.33**).

Fig. 4.33

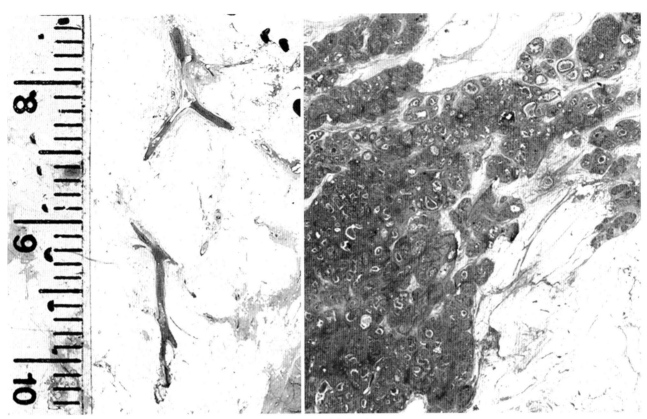

Fig. 4.34 (Reprinted from reference 7 with permission of the publisher.)

Cancer in situ may also develop within the ducts, with or without involving TDLUs. The malignant cells of such carcinomas are still able to maintain the normal ductal architecture in many cases. The involved ducts are dilated, but their number and the number of their branches are normal (**Fig. 4.34**, left image). The most aggressive cases of DCIS are characterized by cancer-filled, duct-like structures close to each other. Their number is much higher than the normal, anatomically expected number of ducts. The malignant cells in such carcinomas are no longer able to maintain the normal ductal–lobular architecture because of a block of the genetic program of alveolar switch, which is essential for forming TDLUs. Instead, irregular duct-like structures are formed with a present but malfunctioning myoepithelial cell layer surrounded by a defective basement membrane. Similarly to the newly formed ducts in the embryo, these duct-like structures are surrounded by a thick layer of a protein called tenascin C. One such duct-like structure is illustrated in **Fig. 4.35** showing c-erb-B2 expressing cancer cells (stained red), brown dots corresponding to the nuclei of the myoepithelial cells, and a thick layer of tenascin C (also brown). This phenomenon is designated as *neoductgenesis* (**Fig. 4.34**, right image) and is considered to be a biologically intermediate lesion between clearly in situ and clearly invasive cancers.

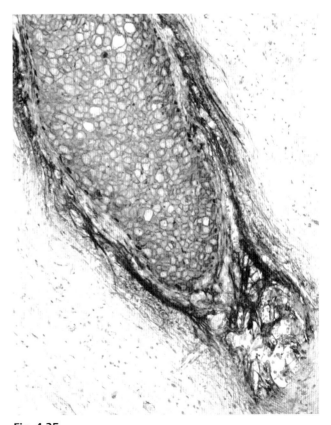

Fig. 4.35

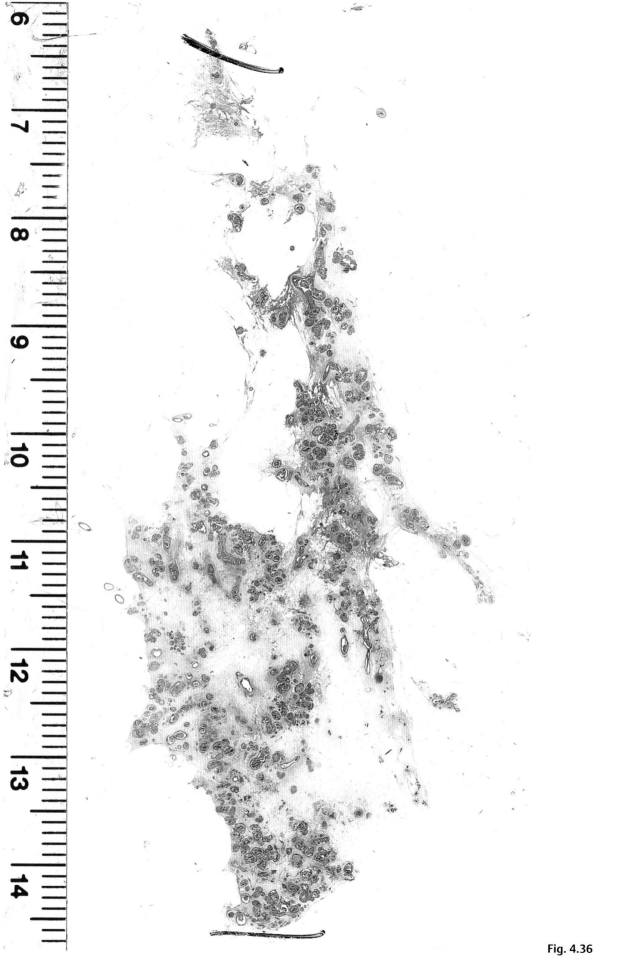

Fig. 4.36

Fig. 4.36 also shows a case of DCIS grade III with signs of neoductgenesis (increased number of ducts compared with the anatomically expected number). Periductal lymphocytic infiltration (**Figs. 4.37** and **4.38**) is often present around the newly formed ducts and represents an indirect sign of neoductgenesis, as well as periductal tenascin accumulation (**Figs. 4.39** and **4.40**). DCIS involving the ducts, especially those with signs of neoductgenesis, is often extensive.

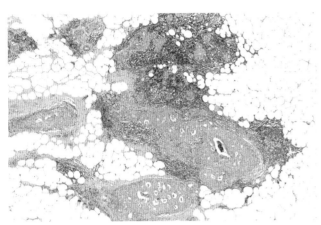

Fig. 4.37

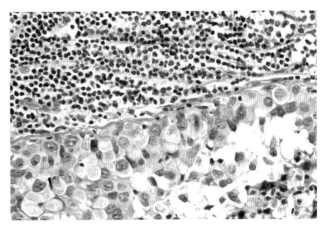

Fig. 4.38

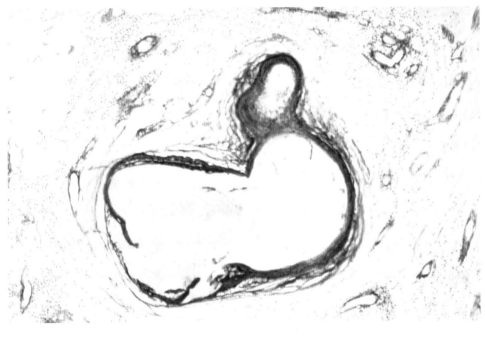

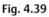

Fig. 4.39

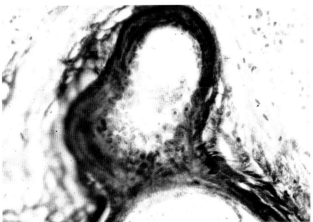

Fig. 4.40

The prognostically different categories of DCIS differ from each other not only in histological grade (I, II, and III) but also in their *extent* and *distribution*. Because tumor size is defined by the largest diameter of the largest invasive focus, DCIS is measured by its extent.

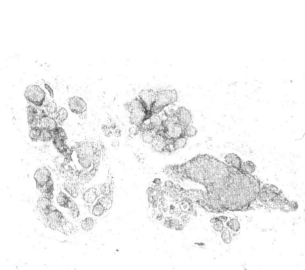

Fig. 4.41

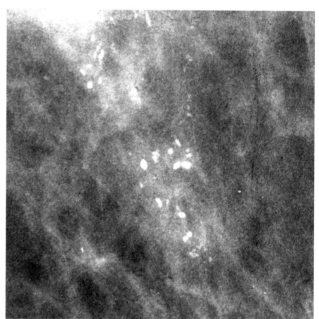

Fig. 4.43

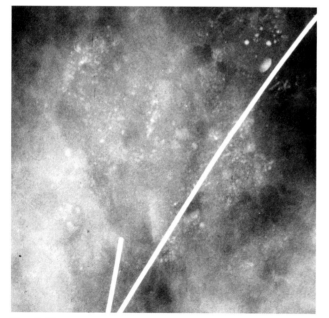

Fig. 4.42

Fig. 4.44

DCIS grade I typically appears as multiple, somewhat dilated and distorted lobules filled with cancer cells (**Fig. 4.41**). It may contain psammoma body–like microcalcifications. The typical mammographic appearance in these cases is the presence of clustered powdery microcalcifications (**Fig. 4.42**). This grade of DCIS may be *extensive and multifocal.*

DCIS grade II usually grows in an extremely dilated TDLU (**Fig. 4.43**). Central necrosis is often present with or without microcalcifications. The calcifications are amorphous and of the broken-needle type (**Fig. 4.44**). This DCIS is of *limited extent, often unifocal*, or less significantly multifocal.

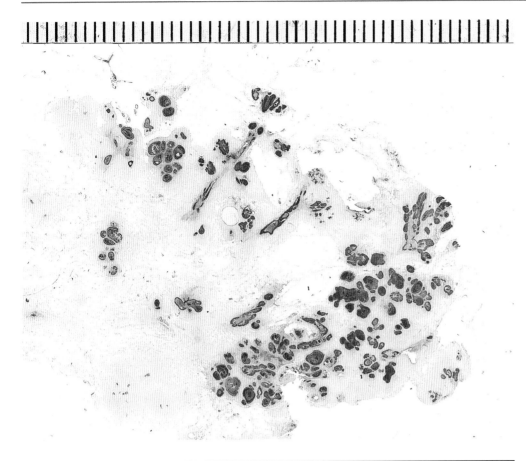

Fig. 4.45

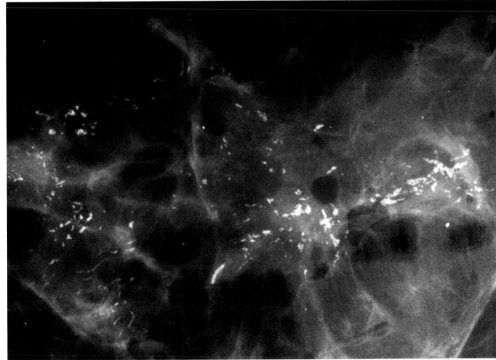

Fig. 4.46

DCIS grade III often originates in larger ducts and has the potential to involve preformed ducts and lobules, and to form new ducts (**Fig. 4.45**). This grade of DCIS often contains "casting type" microcalcifications (**Fig. 4.46**). DCIS grade III is often *extensive* and *diffuse.*

Taking into account all breast carcinomas with DCIS (purely in situ tumors and invasive carcinomas having a DCIS component), half of the cases of DCIS grade III and about a quarter of the cases of DCIS grade I and II are calcified. Although uncalcified DCIS may be detected on magnetic resonance imaging (especially if it is of grade III), grades I and II DCIS without calcifications are one of the leading causes of discrepancies between radiologically and histologically determined disease extent.

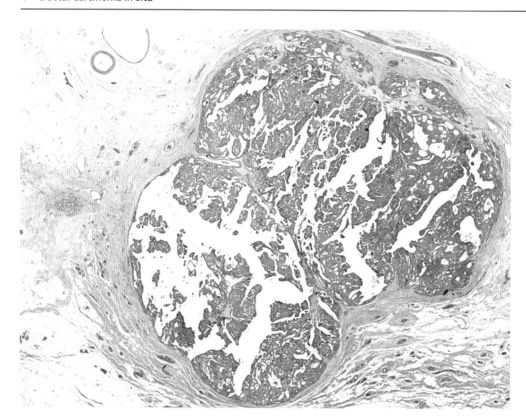

Fig. 4.47

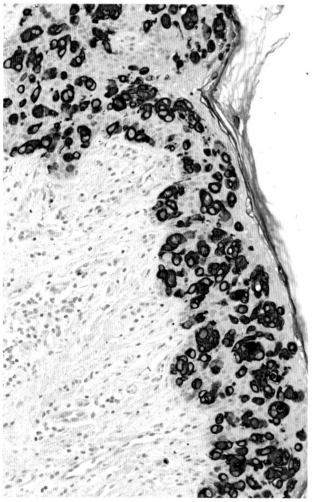

Fig. 4.48

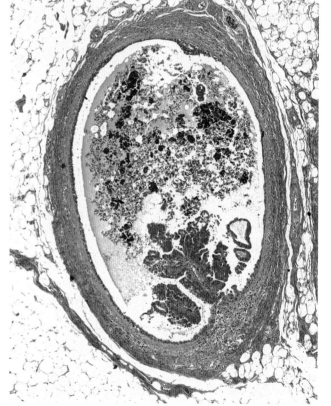

Fig. 4.49

Most cases of DCIS are nonpalpable and asymptomatic and are detected by finding microcalcifications at mammographic screening. However, approximately 20% of cases of DCIS, the so-called special types, are clinically detectable displaying the following:

–   A palpable cystic tumor ("encapsulated" or "intracystic" papillary carcinoma, **Fig. 4.47**) (see also Chapter 6)

–   A chronic, eczema-like skin lesion in the region of the nipple/areola (Paget disease, **Fig. 4.48**, cytokeratin CAM 5.2 staining)

–   Nipple discharge (intraductal papilloma with DCIS, see Chapter 6, or the so-called apocrine papillary DCIS, **Fig. 4.49**)

–   A palpable lesion appearing as architectural distortion on the mammogram (so-called tumor-forming DCIS, see case 6 in Chapter 10)

–   Solid papillary carcinoma (**Fig. 4.50**), which is often palpable and characterized by an attenuated or absent myoepithelial layer

–   So-called intraductal papillary carcinoma, which may also cause nipple discharge and which is classified as a special form of in situ cancer despite the total absence of myoepithelial cells (**Figs. 4.51** and **4.52**, smooth-muscle actin stain marking cells belonging to a vessel)

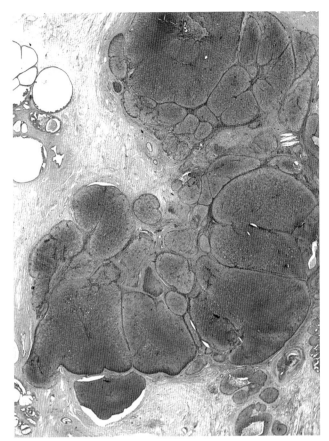

Fig. 4.50

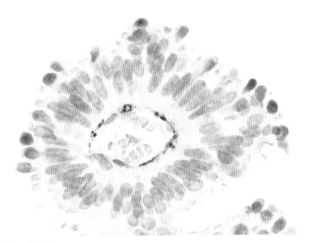

Fig. 4.52

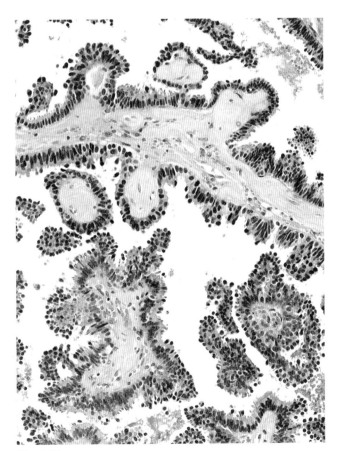

Fig. 4.51

Unlike the borderline lesions discussed in Chapter 3, DCIS grade I is a precursor lesion, in which invasive cancer may develop in the same breast after a period of several years. The prognosis in these cases is usually very good.

DCIS grade III is often a highly aggressive lesion with recurrences even after a seemingly radical excision. Extensive invasive recurrences may develop over a short period. Even if the invasive component is microscopic or undetectable, the prognosis may be unfavorable.

The prognosis of DCIS grade II is intermediate.

The special types of DCIS generally have a good prognosis, with the exception of Paget disease, which is usually a grade III lesion.

Conclusions

DCIS is a very heterogeneous group of diseases, most often detected by mammography. The heterogeneous nature is reflected in characteristic presentations on the mammogram. The histologic appearance varies in cell type, growth pattern, presence of necrosis, nuclear grade, and extent and distribution. Heterogeneity is also often observed within the same tumor.

The most important role of the pathologist in making the diagnosis of DCIS is correct classification, especially recognizing the aggressive forms that need immediate therapeutic intervention and careful follow-up. In a practical approach, delineation of the special types (detected most often clinically) from the rest of in situ carcinomas, detected by finding microcalcifications on the mammograms, should be the first step. The latter types should then be categorized as those involving the TDLUs and those involving mainly the larger ducts. Cases of DCIS involving the TDLUs are either unifocal or multifocal, whereas those involving the larger ducts are diffuse either with or without signs of neoductgenesis. Careful assessment of the extent of disease and the tumor grade is essential.

For a successful pathological workup, it is essential to do the following:

- Correlate the histological and radiological findings.

- Use a simple and reproducible grading system.

- Use the large-section technique because DCIS often extends beyond the area of the microcalcifications.

Bibliography

1. Faverly DRG, Burgers L, Bult P, Holland R. Three dimensional imaging of mammary ductal carcinoma in situ: clinical implications. Semin Diagn Pathol 1994;11(3):193–198
2. Consensus conference on the classification of ductal carcinoma in situ. Hum Pathol 1997;28(11):1221–1225
3. Shoker BS, Sloane JP. DCIS grading schemes and clinical implications. Histopathology 1999;35(5):393–400
4. Silverstein MJ, Lagios MD, Craig PH, et al. A prognostic index for ductal carcinoma in situ of the breast. Cancer 1996;77(11):2267–2274
5. Tot T. DCIS, cytokeratins, and the theory of the sick lobe. Virchows Arch 2005;447(1):1–8
6. Tot T, Tabár L. Mammographic-pathologic correlation of ductal carcinoma in situ of the breast using two- and three-dimensional large histologic sections. Semin Breast Dis 2005;8(3):144–151
7. Tot T. The subgross morphology of the normal and pathologically altered breast tissue. In: Suri J, Rangayyan R, eds. Recent Advances in Breast Imaging, Mammography, and Computer-Aided Diagnosis of Breast Cancer. Bellingham, WA: SPIE Press; 2006:1– 49
8. Castellano I, Marchiò C, Tomatis M, et al. Micropapillary ductal carcinoma in situ of the breast: an inter-institutional study. Mod Pathol 2010;23(2):260–269
9. Tabár L, Tot T, Dean PB. Breast Cancer. Early Detection with Mammography. Casting Type Calcifications: Sign of a Subtype with Deceptive Features. New York, NY: Thieme; 2007
10. Tabár L, Tot T, Dean PB. Early Detection with Mammography: Crushed Stone-Like Calcifications: The Most Frequent Malignant Type. New York, NY: Thieme; 2008

Chapter 5

The Most Common Types of Invasive Breast Carcinoma

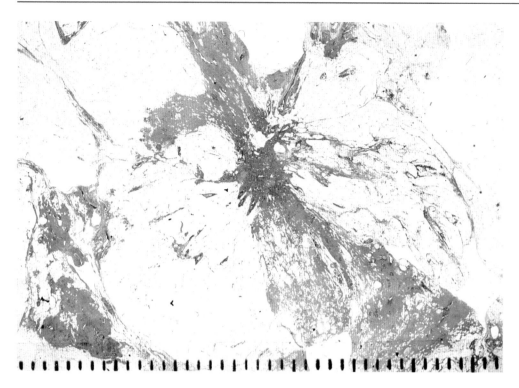

Fig. 5.1

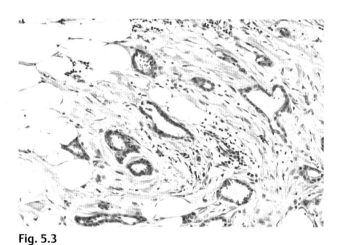

Fig. 5.3

Tubular carcinoma is a slow-growing, stellate tumor with stromal desmoplasia (**Fig. 5.1**). The typical mammographic appearance is a small stellate density with a central tumor mass ("white star") (**Fig. 5.2**).

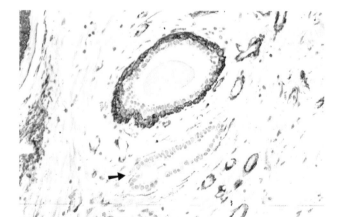

Fig. 5.4

Diagnostic Criteria

More than 90% of the tumor has tubular structures with the following traits:

- Angulated and irregular (**Fig. 5.3**)
- Composed of only one thin layer of epithelial cells
- Absence of myoepithelium (given the single layer of epithelial cells) (**Fig. 5.4**, arrow)

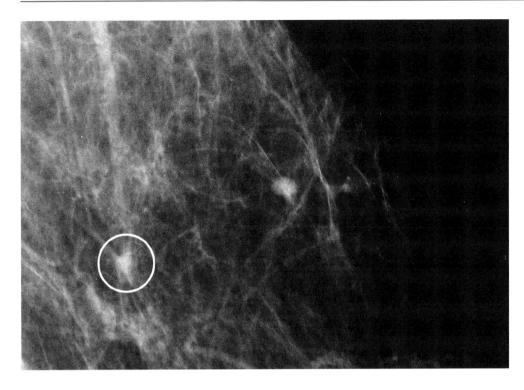

Fig. 5.2

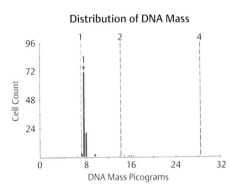

Fig. 5.5

Distribution of DNA Mass

Cell Count

DNA Mass Picograms

Cell Classes
Display: 12 45

First Peak
Mass: 7.8 pg.
DNA Index: 1.09
Area: 73.7 µ²
Cells: 72
Second Peak
Mass: 0.0 pg.
DNA Index: 0.00
Area: 0.0 µ²
Cells: 0

Field Count: 14
Total Cell Count: 104
Cells Displayed: 104

Tubular carcinoma may be multifocal. Structures of ductal carcinoma in situ (DCIS) grade I are regularly present in the tumor. In these cases the mammographic image is multiple stellate tumors bridged together; within the bridge the in situ carcinoma is found at histology. Tubular carcinoma is regularly diploid (**Fig. 5.5**), is estrogen-receptor positive (**Fig. 5.6**), and has an excellent prognosis.

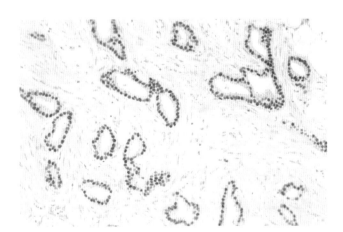

Fig. 5.6

Differential Diagnosis

1. Radial scar (see also Chapter 6)

   a. Usually not palpable

   b. Typical mammographic picture of a "black star"

   c. Presence of myoepithelium

2. Microglandular adenosis

   a. Regular, round glands (absence of lobulocentricity and myoepithelium)

3. Invasive ductal carcinoma no special type (NST)

   a. Contains less than 90% tubular structures

Mucinous carcinoma is a mucin-producing, slow-growing tumor with a favorable prognosis. Mammographically, it usually appears as a circular or oval, ill-defined, low-density tumor mass (**Fig. 5.7**).

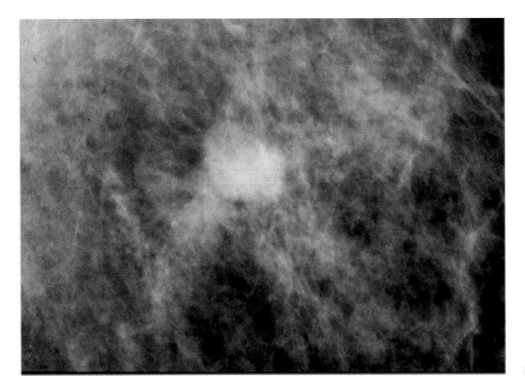

Fig. 5.7

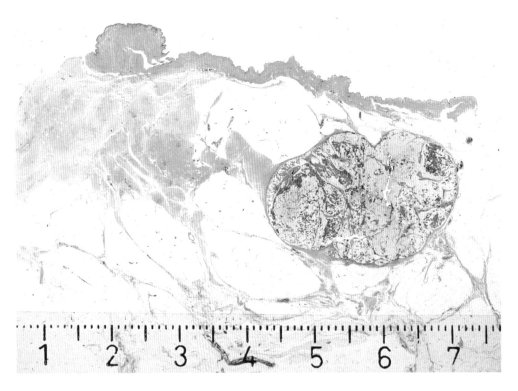

Fig. 5.8

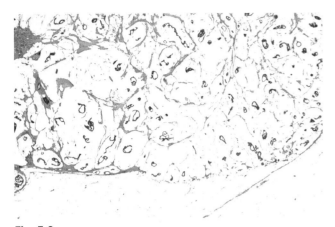

Fig. 5.9

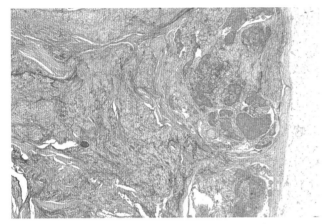

Fig. 5.10

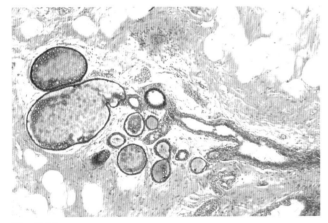

Fig. 5.11

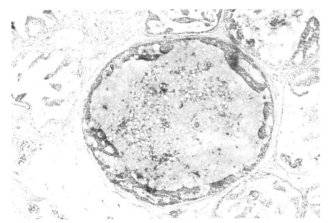

Fig. 5.12

Diagnostic Criteria

- The tumor is macroscopically well circumscribed and gelatinous (**Fig. 5.8**).

- At least 90% of the tumor is composed of mucin, containing small groups of well-differentiated tumor cells (**Figs. 5.9** and **5.10**, Alcian Blue staining).

A tumor fulfilling these criteria has an excellent prognosis. However, mucinous carcinoma often exhibits obvious intratumoral heterogeneity (see Chapter 10, Case 1), which may have prognostic implications.

Differential Diagnosis

1. Mucin-containing lobules (**Fig. 5.11**, Alcian Blue staining), dilated ducts, mucocele and mucinous DCIS (**Fig. 5.12**, Alcian Blue staining)

2. Ductal carcinoma with mucinous component

   a. Poorly circumscribed, often stellate

   b. More cellular

   c. Often less well-differentiated tumor cells

   Ductal carcinomas with a mucinous component do not share the favorable prognosis of purely mucinous carcinomas.

3. Invasive micropapillary carcinoma (see Chapter 6)

Medullary carcinoma is usually a rapidly growing, round or oval, well-circumscribed tumor appearing in younger patients. Mammographically, ultrasonographically, or on magnetic resonance imaging (MRI) (**Fig. 5.13**), a circumscribed, solid, round, or oval density is observed.

Macroscopically and histologically the tumor is well circumscribed, relatively soft, and often lobulated (**Fig. 5.14**).

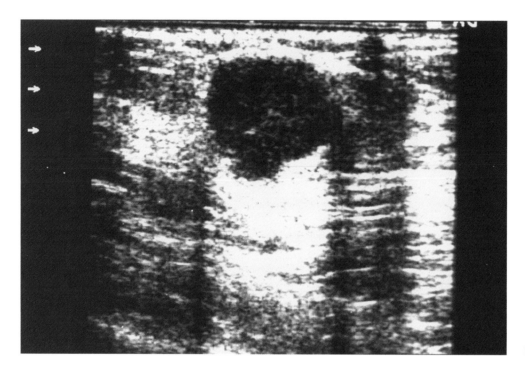

Fig. 5.13

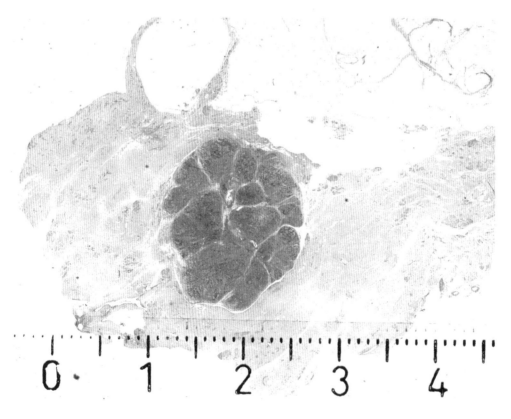

Fig. 5.14

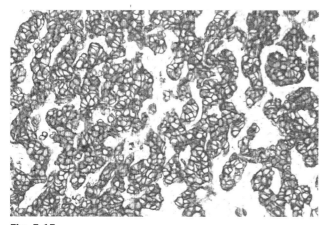

Fig. 5.15

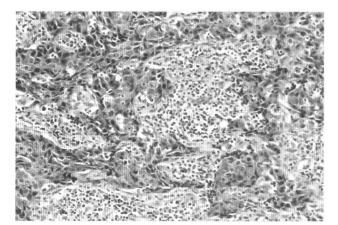

Fig. 5.16

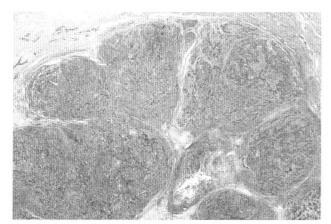

Fig. 5.17

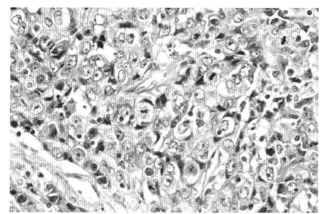

Fig. 5.18

Diagnostic Criteria

– Syncytial growth pattern (**Fig. 5.15**, cytokeratin CAM 5.2 immunostaining)

– Intensive lymphoplasmacytic infiltrate in the stroma (**Fig. 5.16**)

– Noninfiltrating ("pushing") tumor border (**Fig. 5.17**)

– Highly atypical tumor cells (**Fig. 5.18**)

An in situ component and stromal desmoplasia are not features of this tumor.

Tumors with all four criteria are "typical medullary carcinomas" and have a somewhat more favorable prognosis when compared with ductal carcinomas of the same size and grade. "Atypical medullary carcinomas" with only some medullary features (e.g., infiltrating tumor border as in **Fig. 5.19**) share an unfavorable prognosis with their ductal counterparts.

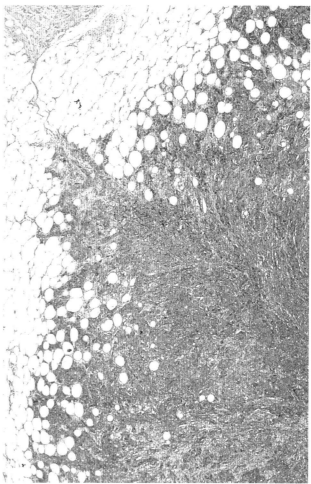

Fig. 5.19

Differential Diagnosis

1. Fibroadenoma (see Chapter 6)

Invasive lobular carcinomas are a heterogeneous group of tumors.

Diagnostic Criteria

– Cell files, one or two cells thick (**Fig. 5.20**)

– And/or small, monomorphous tumor cells, often with intracytoplasmic vacuoles (**Fig. 5.21**)

The criteria have alternative characteristics: tumors composed of cell files classify as lobular even if the tumor cells are larger, more polymorphous, and lacking vacuolization ("pleomorphic variant of lobular breast carcinoma," **Figs. 5.22** and **5.29**). The tumor cells may also exhibit phenotypic variations such as a histiocytoid (**Fig. 5.23**) or a signet-ring (**Fig. 5.24**) appearance.

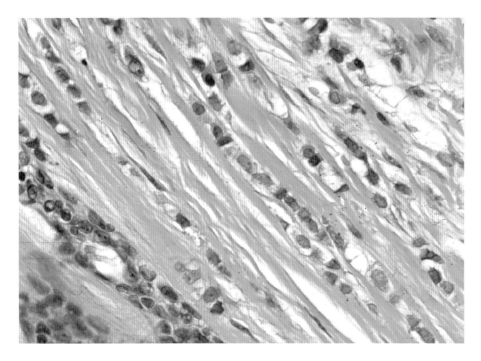

Fig. 5.20

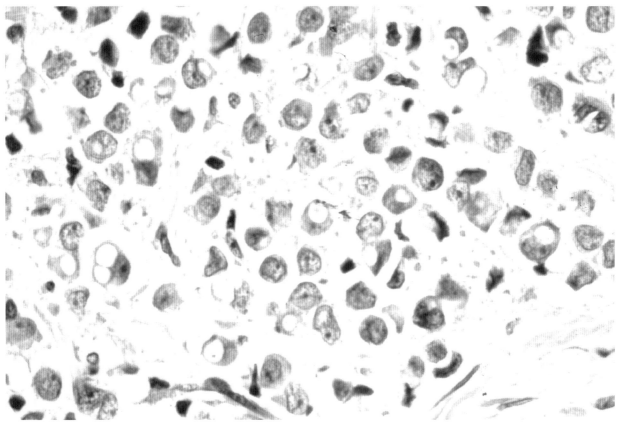

Fig. 5.21

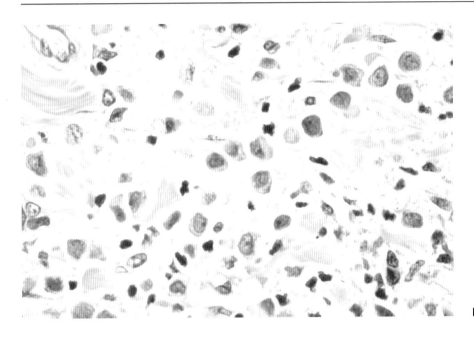

Fig. 5.22

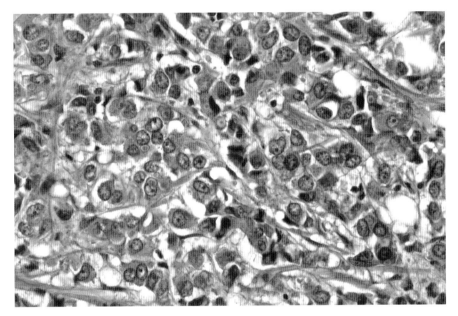

Fig. 5.23

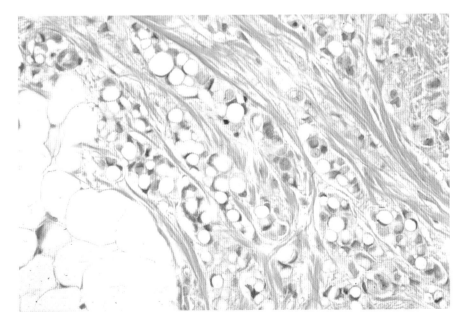

Fig. 5.24

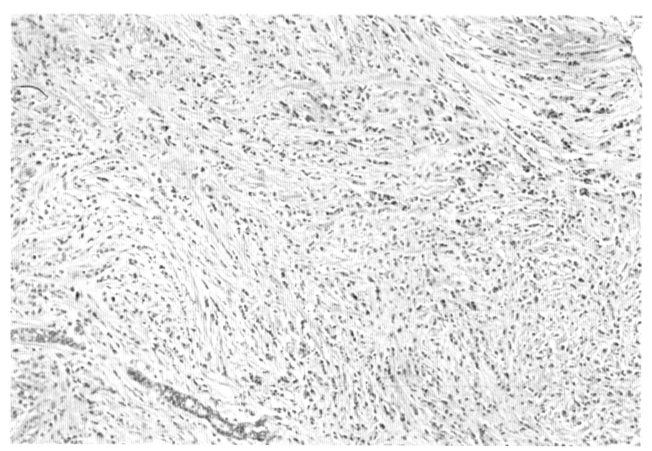

Fig. 5.25

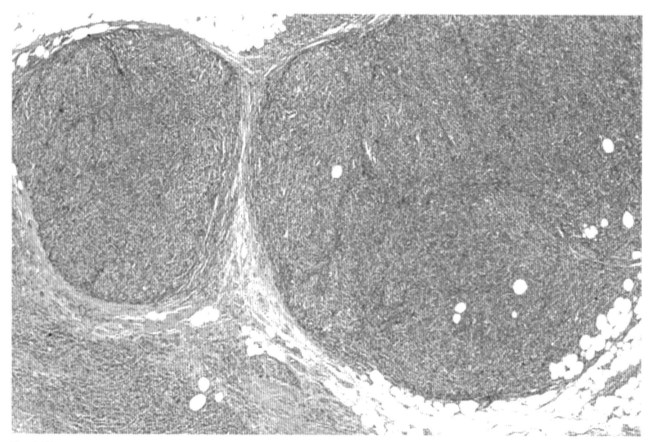

Fig. 5.26

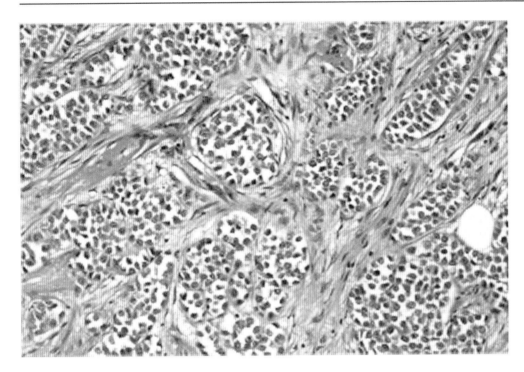

Fig. 5.27

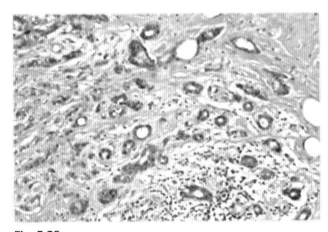

Fig. 5.28

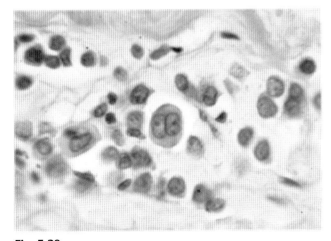

Fig. 5.29

More importantly, if the cells are of the lobular type, the tumors are classified as lobular carcinoma even if the cells are not growing in cell files.

1. Tumors fulfilling both criteria for lobular carcinoma are called invasive lobular carcinoma of the classic type. These tumors are composed of files of small monomorphous cells (Fig. 5.25). The classic invasive lobular carcinoma is often a diffuse, spider's web–like lesion on the mammogram.

2. A solid variant of invasive lobular carcinoma is composed of typical small monomorphous cells that grow in large solid nodules (Fig. 5.26). The solid invasive lobular carcinoma tends to be a circular/oval-shaped tumor mass on the mammogram.

3. An alveolar variant of invasive lobular carcinoma contains typical cells grouped in small solid nests of 10 to 20 tumor cells (Fig. 5.27) and is often occult mammographically.

4. A tubulolobular variant is composed partly of tubular structures and partly cell files of typical cells (Fig. 5.28). This variant has a better prognosis than the other subgroups. The tubulolobular carcinoma has a stellate appearance with a central tumor mass surrounded by straight spiculations.

5. Mixed examples of invasive lobular carcinoma containing more than one of the aforementioned variants are usual.

Ductal carcinomas may contain areas of classical invasive lobular carcinoma or its variants. Mixed carcinomas with clearly separated ductal and lobular components also exist. To classify a tumor as invasive lobular carcinoma, at least 90% of the tumor should exhibit one of the patterns described above.

As already mentioned, invasive lobular carcinoma may form a stellate tumor body (**Figs. 5.30** and **5.31**). Frequently, the classic or the mixed types of invasive lobular carcinoma grow diffusely, extensively permeate the normal tissue, and form a spider's web–like structure without a well-formed tumor body (**Fig. 5.32**). These tumors may grow to several centimeters before causing any mammographic abnormality. They may be detected clinically as palpable lesions or be found by ultrasonography or MRI. The diffuse type of invasive lobular carcinoma comprises approximately 75% of all diffuse invasive carcinomas having unfavorable prognosis (see Chapter 9).

The solid and mixed lobular carcinomas can form well-circumscribed, solid tumors with easily assessable size and limited extent. Even in these cases, multifocality often appears.

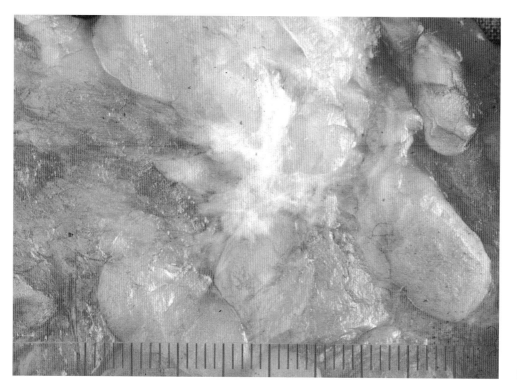

Fig. 5.30

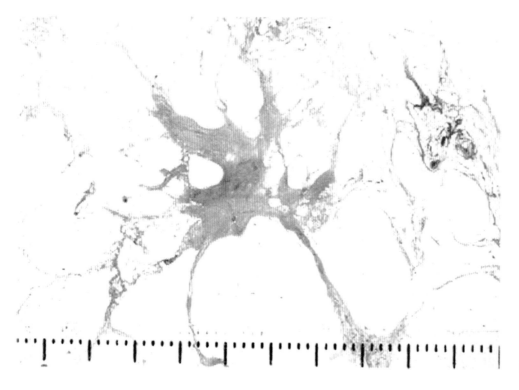

Fig. 5.31

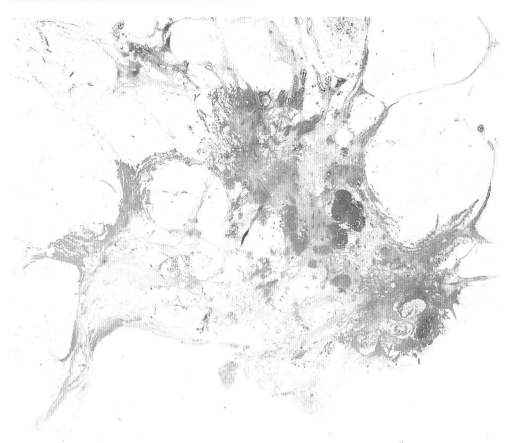

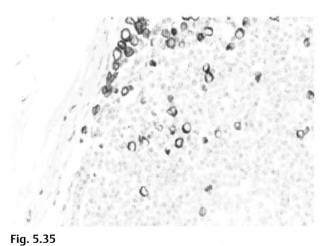

Fig. 5.32

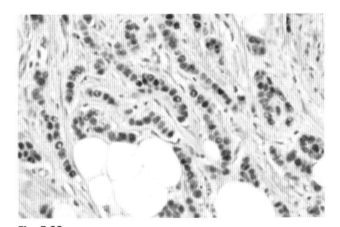

Fig. 5.33

Detection of a primary and metastatic lobular carcinoma can be very difficult, even on histology. Immunohistochemistry may be helpful in detecting the small, dispersed cells of these tumors. The cells are usually estrogen-receptor positive (Fig. 5.33) and react with epithelial markers (Figs. 5.34 and 5.35). As mentioned in Chapter 3, most in situ and invasive lobular carcinomas are either negative for E-cadherin or show reduced expression of this cell surface protein.

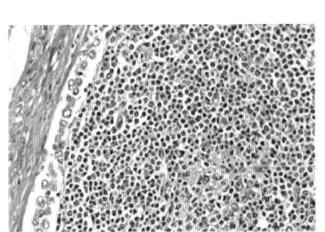

Fig. 5.34

Fig. 5.35

Distribution of breast cancer cases by histological tumor type

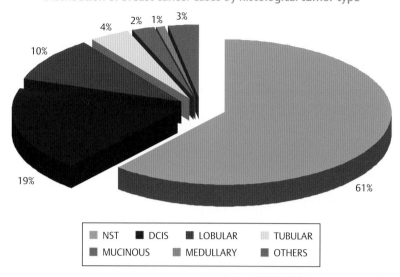

▨ NST	■ DCIS	■ LOBULAR	▧ TUBULAR
▨ MUCINOUS	▨ MEDULLARY	■ OTHERS	

Fig. 5.36 (own results, 1995–98)

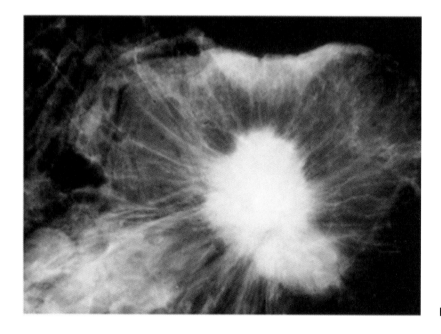

Fig. 5.37

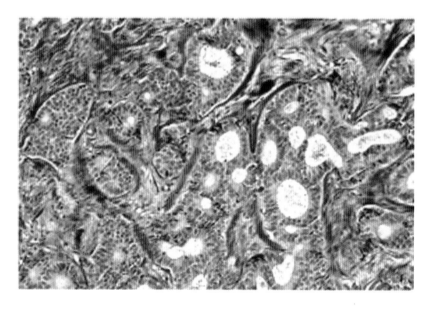

Fig. 5.38

This chapter is restricted to the most usual types of invasive breast carcinomas, despite the existence of many other rare tumor types. Although recognition and proper classification of these rare tumors may represent a challenge for the pathologist, the other members of the breast team are more interested in the usual morphological prognostic parameters (size, distribution, extent, and grade), even in these cases. For practical purposes, it is more important to find the similarities between the carcinoma cases than to find minor histological differences.

As seen in **Fig. 5.36**, most of the invasive breast carcinomas do not fulfill the criteria of any of the breast carcinomas of special type. They belong to the category of invasive (ductal) breast carcinoma of "no special type" (NST) (**Figs. 5.37** and **5.38**), a large and heterogeneous group of adenocarcinomas containing more than 60% of all breast malignancies. This prognostically heterogeneous tumor group needs to be stratified by use of morphological prognostic factors (see Chapter 9).

Conclusions

By restrictive use of morphological criteria, special types of mammary carcinomas can be diagnosed. Tubular and mucinous carcinomas with typical histological patterns in at least 90% of the tumor have an excellent prognosis. Typical medullary carcinomas have a better prognosis than their ductal counterparts. It is important to recognize lobular carcinomas because of the many variations of this tumor type and their tendency to be more extensive than suspected on the mammogram. Most of the invasive carcinomas, however, belong to a single large and heterogeneous group of invasive breast carcinomas of no special type which has to be stratified by the use of morphological prognostic parameters.

Bibliography

1. Chinyama CN, Davies JD. Mammary mucinous lesions: congeners, prevalence and important pathological associations. Histopathology 1996;29(6):533–539
2. Toikkanen S, Pylkkänen L, Joensuu H. Invasive lobular carcinoma of the breast has better short- and long-term survival than invasive ductal carcinoma. Br J Cancer 1997;76(9):1234–1240
3. Pedersen L. Medullary carcinoma of the breast. APMIS Suppl 1997;75:1–31
4. Tot T. The role of cytokeratins 20 and 7 and estrogen receptor analysis in separation of metastatic lobular carcinoma of the breast and metastatic signet ring cell carcinoma of the gastrointestinal tract. APMIS 2000;108(6):467–472
5. Tot T. The cytokeratin profile of medullary carcinoma of the breast. Histopathology 2000;37(2):175–181
6. Tabár L, Vitak B, Chen HH, et al. The Swedish Two-County Trial twenty years later. Updated mortality results and new insights from long-term follow-up. Radiol Clin North Am 2000;38(4):625–651
7. Tot T. The diffuse type of invasive lobular carcinoma of the breast: morphology and prognosis. Virchows Arch 2003;443(6):718–724
8. Tavassoli FA, Eusebi V. Tumors of the Mammary Gland. AFIP Atlas of Tumor Pathology Series 4, vol 10. Washington, DC: American Registry of Pathology; 2009
9. Lakhani SR, Ellis IO, Schnitt SJ, et al. eds. WHO Classification of Tumors of the Breast. Lyon, France: International Agency for Research on Cancer; 2012

Chapter 6

The Most Common Benign Breast Lesions and their Borderline and Malignant Counterparts

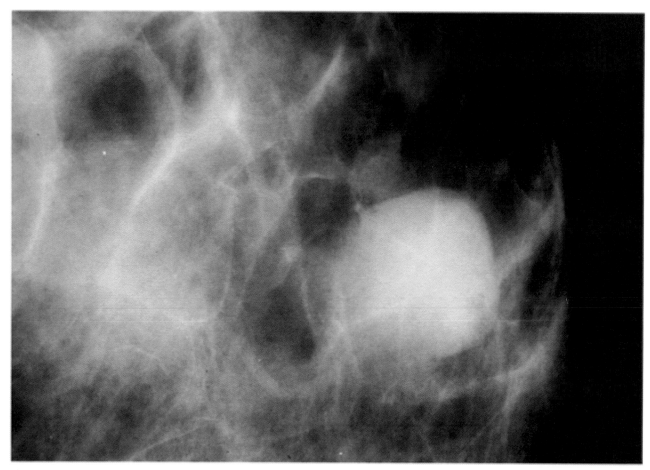

Fig. 6.1

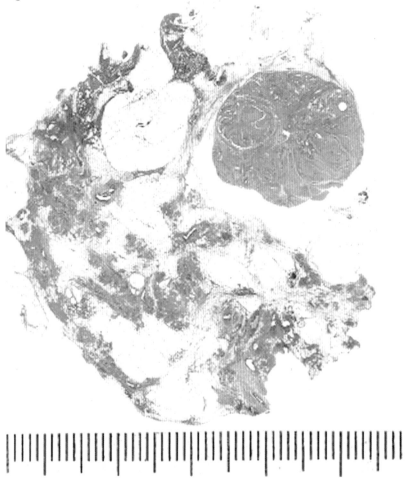

Fig. 6.2

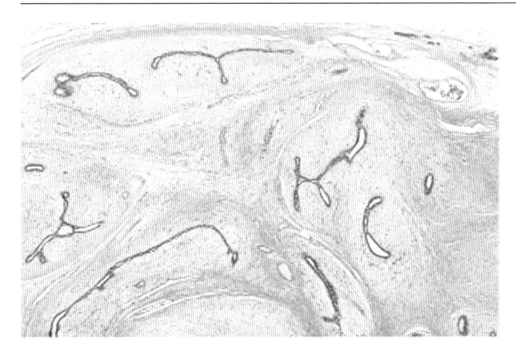

Fig. 6.3

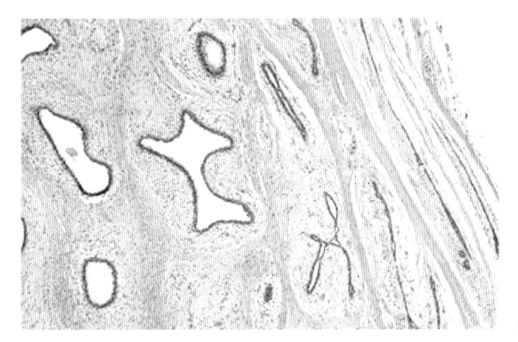

Fig. 6.4

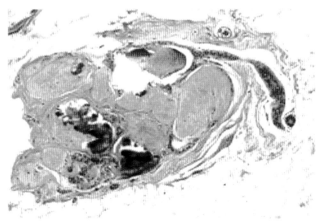

Fig. 6.5

Fibroadenoma (**Figs. 6.1** and **6.2**) is a very common benign epithelial-stromal tumor, mainly containing proliferated elements of the intralobular active stroma but also featuring proliferated ducts and acini. The epithelial component is distorted in the so-called intracanalicular variant (**Fig. 6.3**) and more regular in "pericanalicular" fibroadenoma (**Fig. 6.4**). The epithelial component may exhibit hyperplastic or metaplastic changes. The stroma of the younger lesion is mucin-rich and becomes more fibrous over time. Fibroadenoma is usually a palpable lesion, but in approximately 10% of the cases, it is detected on the basis of amorphous stromal microcalcifications (**Fig. 6.5**) seen on the mammogram. Fibroadenoma represents a clinically detectable phase of fibroadenomatoid change (see Chapter 1).

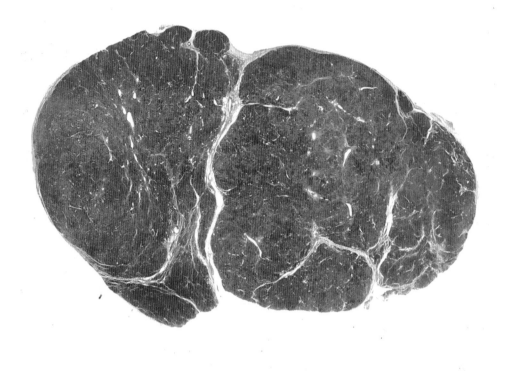

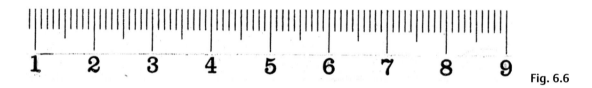

Fig. 6.6

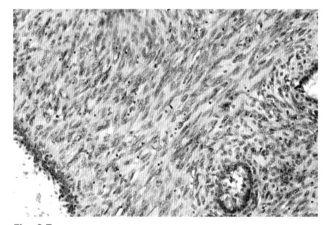

Fig. 6.7

The stroma in a fibroadenoma is poorly cellular and mitotically almost inactive. The "juvenile" variant of fibroadenoma is a more rapidly growing round or oval lesion that has a more cellular stroma with some mitotic figures (Fig. 6.6).

The term *phylloides tumor* designates a group of epithelial-stromal neoplasms with dominating stroma and leaflike structures (Figs. 6.7 and 6.8). The stroma in these lesions is more cellular and mitotically active, even in benign cases. An occurrence of more than 5 mitoses per 10 high-power fields is considered as an indicator of low malignant potential ("phylloides tumor of borderline malignancy") with a tendency to recur. Lesions with obvious stromal cellular atypia and high mitotic activity are rare and malignant. They may contain heterologous stromal components (e.g., liposarcoma, rhabdomyosarcoma, or osteosarcoma).

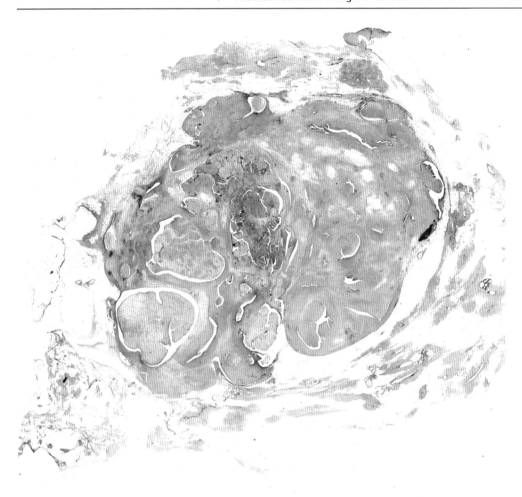

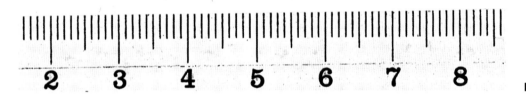

Fig. 6.8

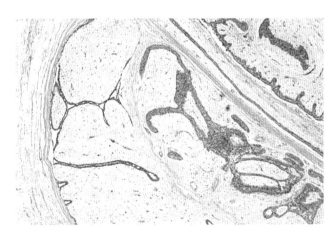

Fig. 6.9

The epithelial component of these tumors may contain foci of lobular carcinoma in situ (LCIS), ductal carcinoma in situ (DCIS) (**Fig. 6.9**), or invasive carcinoma.

The most important issue in this group of lesions is the potential risk of overdiagnosis. In the presence of a growing palpable mass, usually in younger women, a cellular fine-needle aspirate may lead to an erroneous preoperative diagnosis of malignancy. Core biopsy usually rules out the possibility of carcinoma and detects the rare borderline and malignant variants of these tumors.

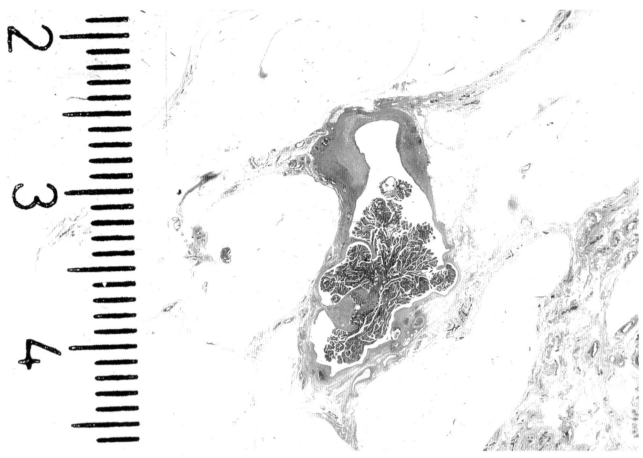

Fig. 6.10

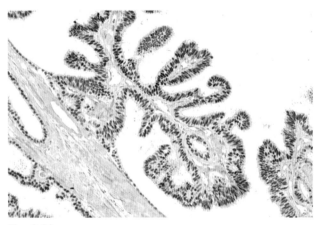

Fig. 6.11

One of the few lesions that often originate outside the terminal ductal-lobular unit (TDLU) is a *papilloma*. It usually develops in larger ducts in the retroareolar area ("central" papilloma) and often causes serous or bloody nipple discharge. "Peripheral" papillomas originate in the TDLUs or smaller ducts and are often multiple. Papillomas are exophytic lesions that fill the lumen of the dilated duct (**Fig. 6.10**) and contain a branching fibrous central core (**Figs. 6.11** and **6.12**).

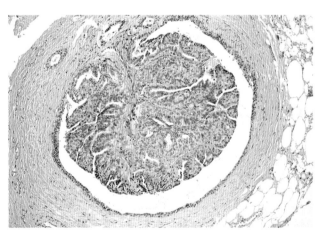

Fig. 6.12

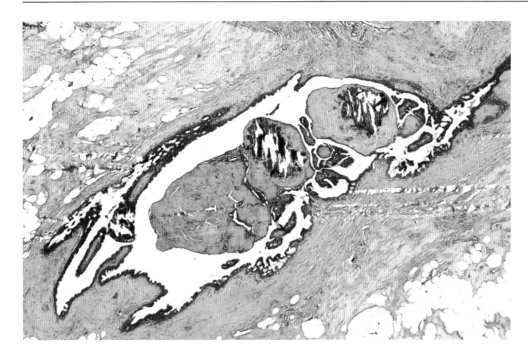

Fig. 6.13

On the mammogram papillomas are usually < 10 mm circular/oval shaped masses, with or without associated calcifications, which can be either coarse or crushed stone–like (**Fig. 6.13**). In case of serous or bloody nipple discharge, galactography or breast MRI are the procedures of choice to detect the cause of discharge, which, in most cases is a benign papilloma (**Fig. 6.14**).

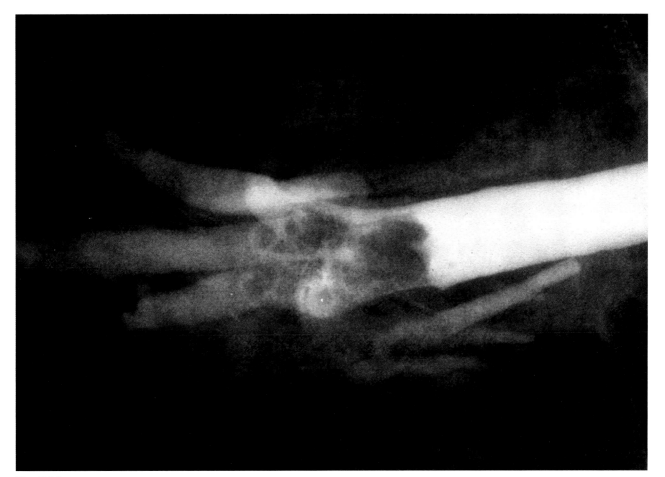

Fig. 6.14

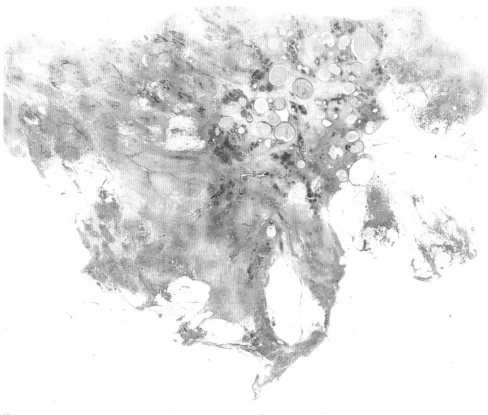

Fig. 6.15

Papillomas may be solitary or multiple. Sometimes in young women multiple papillomas appear in a fibrocystic area of the breast tissue. This is referred to as juvenile papillomatosis (Fig. 6.15).

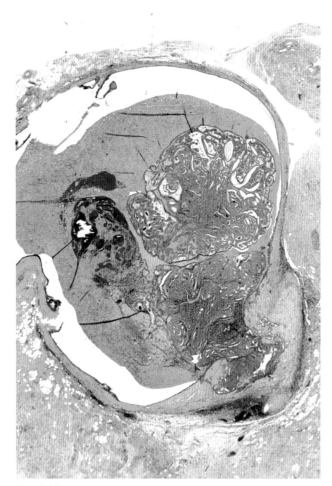

Fig. 6.16

The epithelial component as well as the myoepithelium in papillomas may exhibit a spectrum of metaplastic, hyperplastic, and neoplastic changes resulting in benign, borderline, and malignant categories of the papillary lesions. At the benign end of the spectrum are intraductal papillomas with a single layer of epithelium and a single layer of myoepithelium, but metaplasia or hyperplasia of the epithelium and the myoepithelium frequently occurs. Infarction of papillomas may occur and lead to bloody discharge (Fig. 6.16).

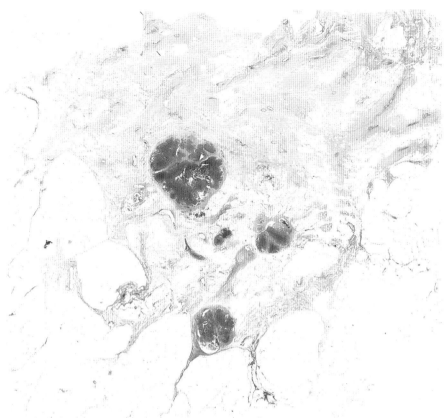

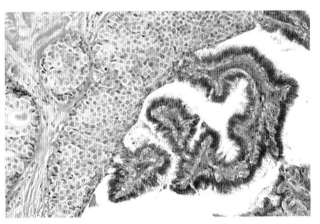

Fig. 6.17

Fig. 6.19

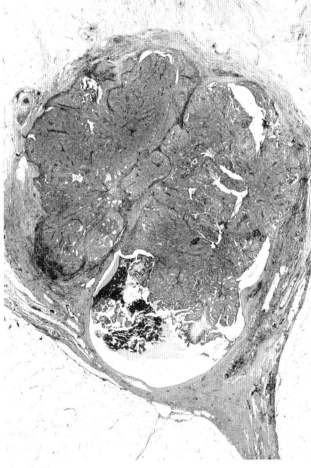

Fig. 6.18

The borderline category of papillary lesions is a heterogeneous group of noninfiltrating tumors with good prognosis (**Figs. 6.17**, **6.18**, and **6.19**). They may contain foci of atypical ductal hyperplasia (ADH), DCIS, or LCIS. Terms such as *atypical papilloma* (if the malignant focus is < 3 mm in diameter) or *malignant papilloma* (if the focus is ≥ 3 mm) have been proposed for diagnostic use in these cases. The diagnostic criteria for hyperplasia, atypical hyperplasia, and carcinoma in situ within the papillomas are the same as those discussed in Chapter 3.

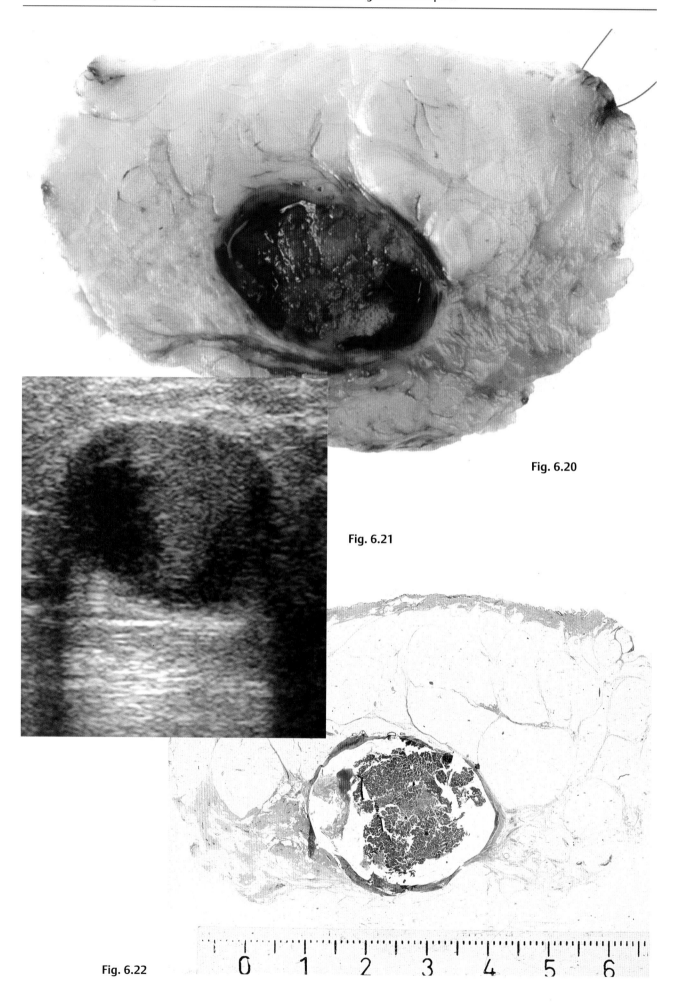

Fig. 6.20

Fig. 6.21

Fig. 6.22

If the duct containing a papillary lesion becomes cystically dilated, the lesion is designated as an intracystic papilloma or encapsulated/intracystic papillary carcinoma. The intracystic papillary carcinoma contains large areas of malignant cells (usually grade I) grouped into papillary structures with a less evident fibrotic core and myoepithelium. Ordinary structures of DCIS in the TDLUs in the vicinity of the intracystic lesion, if present, represent further evidence of malignancy (**Figs. 6.20, 6.21,** and **6.22**). Intracystic papillary tumors appear on the mammogram as solitary or multiple high density circular/oval-shaped tumor masses. Ultrasound examination demonstrates the intracystic papillary growth exquisitely (**Fig. 6.21**), but the differential diagnosis between benign and malignant intracystic tumor requires histologic examination.

The prognostic significance of small areas of invasion in a case of otherwise typical intracystic papillary carcinomas is unknown. If the infiltrative pattern predominates, the tumor is invasive papillary carcinoma, representing a special form of invasive breast carcinomas (**Fig. 6.23**) in which 90% of the tumor has to exhibit a papillary pattern. The papillary pattern may be seen focally in ductal, mucinous, or mixed carcinomas. The invasive micropapillary carcinoma is another rare breast carcinoma of a special type that typically consists of small papillary structures with inverse polarity of the cells (**Fig. 6.24**).

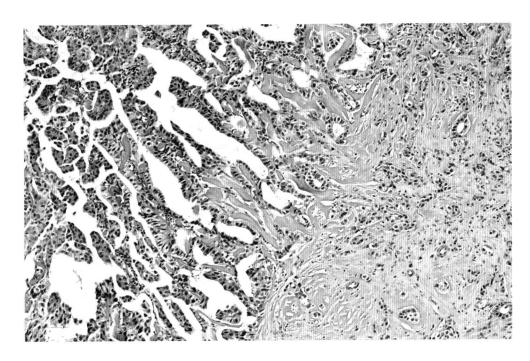

Fig. 6.23

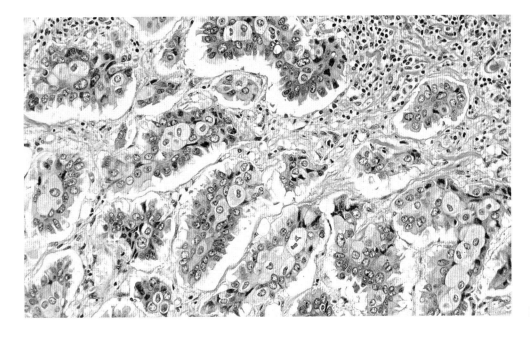

Fig. 6.24

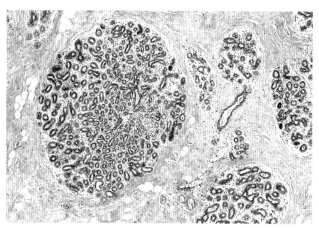

Fig. 6.25

Whereas ductal hyperplasia leads to multilayering of the epithelial cells (see Chapter 3), *adenosis* represents a different form of hyperplasia resulting in increased numbers of acini per lobule, enlargement, and sometimes distortion of lobules. The acini in these lesions retain the normal epithelial monolayer. There are many variations of adenosis according to the architecture and the epithelial cell characteristics. Most of them are restricted to the lobules, but some rare variants do not respect the borders of the lobules.

The most common lobulocentric variants are simple adenosis, sclerosing adenosis, and blunt duct adenosis. Simple adenosis (**Fig. 6.25**) is the prototype of these lesions: an enlarged lobule with an increased number of acini.

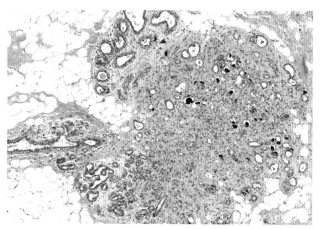

Fig. 6.26

In the very common sclerosing adenosis, the myoepithelium and the stromal cells also proliferate and distort the acini (**Fig. 6.26**). Sometimes on higher microscopic magnification these lesions may resemble an invasive carcinoma (**Figs. 6.27** and **6.28**), which can be ruled out if attention is focused on lobulocentricity of these lesions.

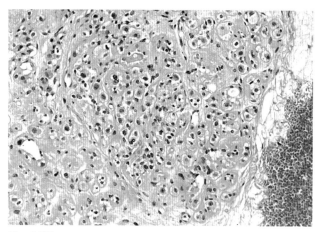

Fig. 6.27

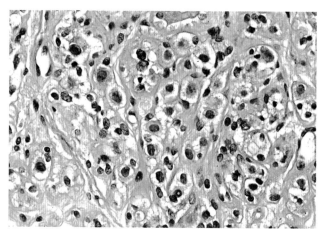

Fig. 6.28

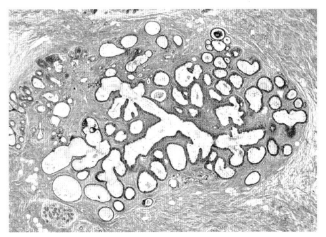

Fig. 6.29

The blunt duct type of adenosis has somewhat dilated acini containing high columnar epithelium (**Fig. 6.29**). In contrast to microcystic involution (**Figs. 1.35** and **1.36**) the number of acini in the lobule is not decreased. This lesion is related to columnar cell change described in Chapter 3.

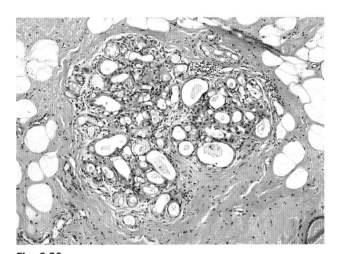

Fig. 6.30

The epithelium in adenosis may exhibit apocrine metaplasia and, rarely, obvious cellular atypia. These variants are designated as apocrine adenosis, atypical adenosis, or, if these cellular changes are combined, atypical apocrine adenosis (**Figs. 6.30, 6.31**, and **6.32**). The biological relevance of these findings is unclear, but there is evidence to support the malignant nature of some of these lesions. Immunohistological staining on myoepithelial markers helps to rule out invasion in most variants of adenosis (**Fig. 6.32**).

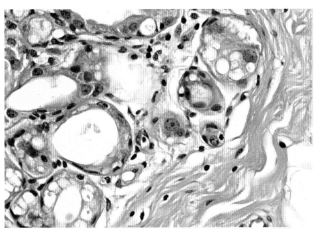

Fig. 6.31

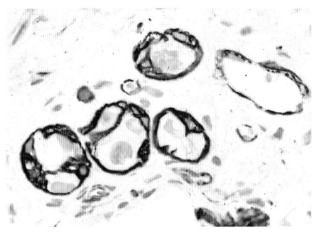

Fig. 6.32

Most often, adenosis represents one of the aberrations of normal development and involution (ANDI), a part of the varying picture of normal breast tissue. However, by coalescence of neighboring enlarged TDLUs, adenosis may form a palpable lesion, the so-called adenosis tumor (**Fig. 6.34**), but this is rare. More often, lobules with adenosis may contain psammoma body–like microcalcifications (**Fig. 6.33**) which, if sufficiently numerous, can be detected on the mammogram as multifocal, lobulocentric powdery calcifications, the same type of microcalcifications as in cases of DCIS grade I (see Chapters 4 and 7).

The hallmark of the common types of adenosis is lobulocentricity. The nonlobulocentric variants (especially the so-called microglandular adenosis consisting of small uniform round acini lacking myoepithelium) always represent a differential diagnostic problem.

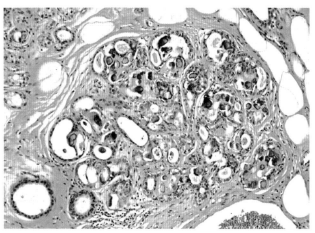

Fig. 6.33

Fig. 6.34

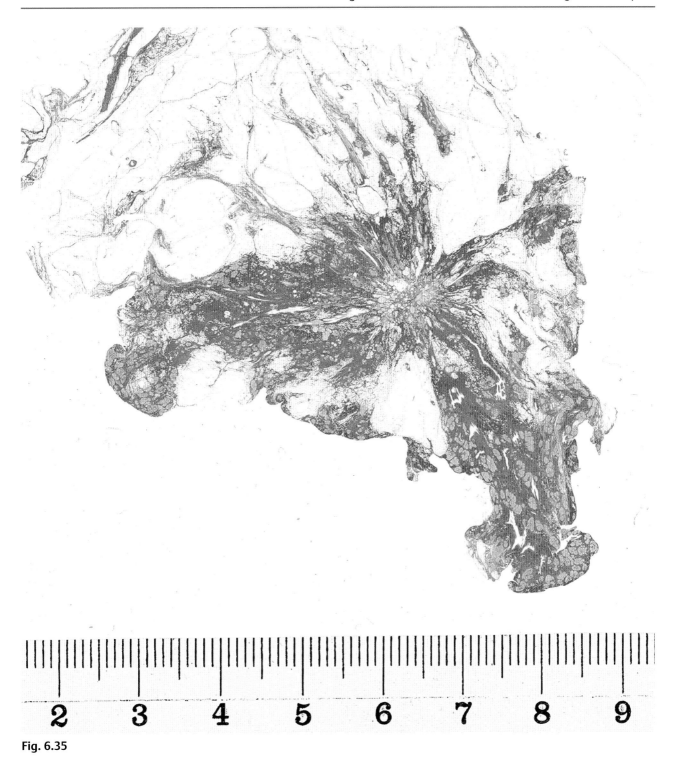

Fig. 6.35

Radial scars are benign lesions with a typical architecture. Centrally they contain a scleroelastic core encircled by a "corona" containing normal lobules or various ANDIs. The radial scars are most often 3- to 5-mm lesions observable only microscopically. Most of the radiologically detected lesions are 15- to 20-mm, nonpalpable, stellate lesions (**Figs. 6.35, 6.36, 6.37, 6.38,** and **6.39**). Sometimes even larger radial scars may develop, which are synonymously called "complex sclerosing lesions."

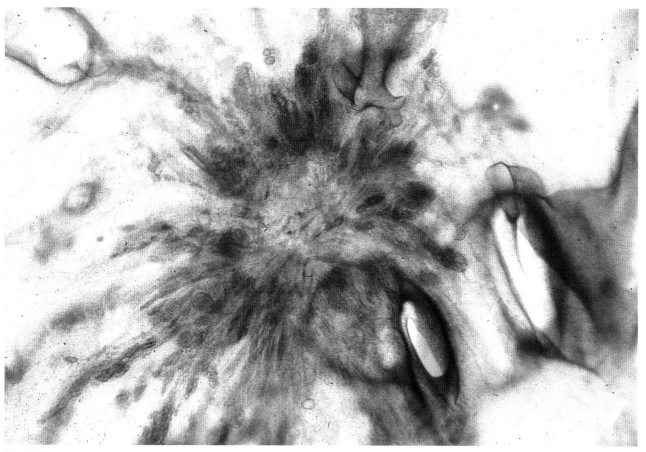

Fig. 6.36

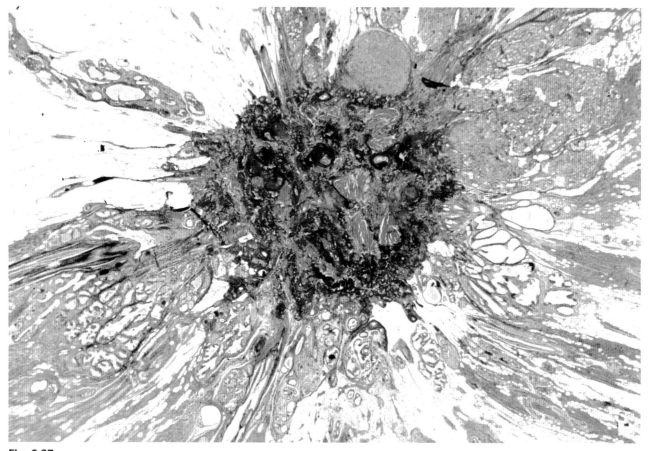

Fig. 6.37

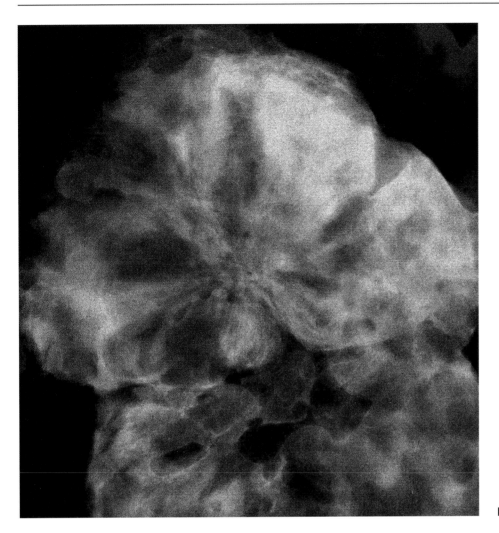

Fig. 6.38

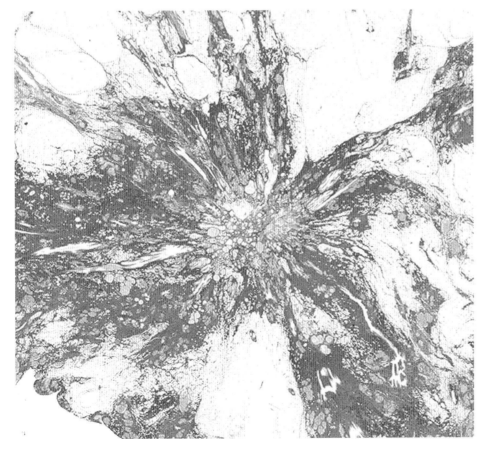

Fig. 6.39

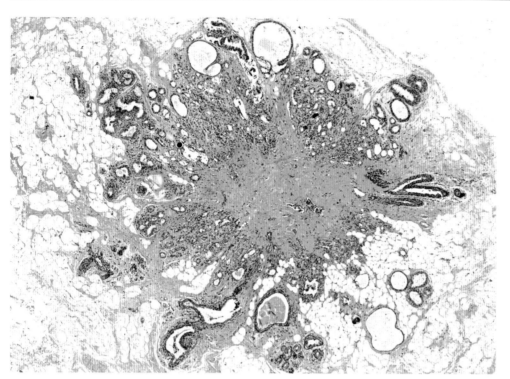

Fig. 6.40

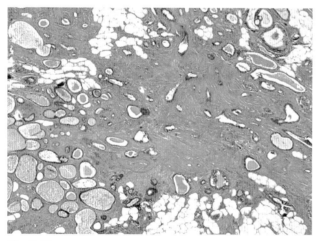

Fig. 6.41

In a considerable proportion of cases, the corona of the radial scars may contain a monotonous population of low-grade cancer cells filling the lobules in a form of atypical lobular hyperplasia (ALH), LCIS, ADH, or DCIS grade I. Because these lesions represent the "borderline area" of malignancy and are usually focal or multifocal, a small sample of the tissue from the corona (e.g., a core biopsy) may not be representative.

Accumulation of elastic fibers in the middle of the lesion usually distorts the preexisting ducts, which may imitate invasion. Because these pseudoinvasive glands lack cellular atypia, the differential diagnostic options include tubular carcinoma or ductal carcinoma NST grade I. The glands in the scleroelastic core of radial scars usually retain the myoepithelial cell layer and do not invade the surrounding fatty tissue (**Figs. 6.40** and **6.41**).

Because they are most often nonpalpable, radial scars are preoperatively detected by mammography. On the

mammogram radial scars lack a solid, central tumor mass, unlike invasive breast cancer. Instead, there may be translucent, oval or circular areas at the central portion of the radiating structure. The architectural distortion consists of radiolucent linear structures, giving it a striking appearance (the so-called black star; **Fig. 6.42**). The radiological appearance of a radial scar differs from invasive carcinomas that usually have a well-developed central, radiopaque tumor mass surrounded by radiopaque, straight spiculations (the so-called white star; **Fig. 6.43**).

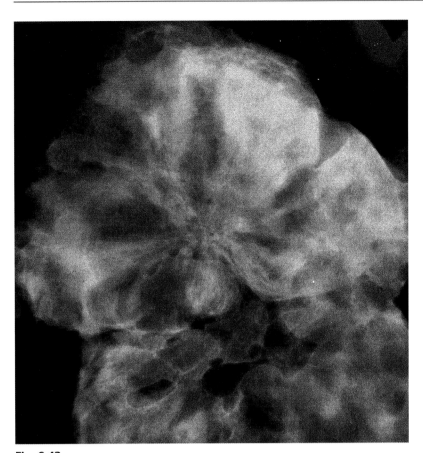

Fig. 6.42

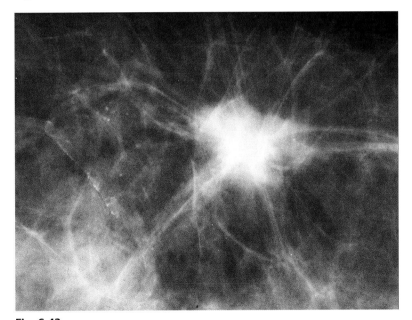

Fig. 6.43

Conclusions

In addition to fibrocystic change (see Chapter 1), fibroadenomas, papillomas, different types of adenosis, and radial scars are the most commonly seen benign breast lesions. A detailed histological workup of these lesions is needed because they may contain foci of malignant cells and because they have rare malignant variants. Some of these lesions have to be included in the differential diagnosis of certain forms of invasive and in situ carcinomas, and some are regarded as a special type of DCIS.

Bibliography

1. Page DL, Salhany KE, Jensen RA, Dupont WD. Subsequent breast carcinoma risk after biopsy with atypia in a breast papilloma. Cancer 1996;78(2):258–266
2. Seidman JD, Ashton M, Lefkowitz M. Atypical apocrine adenosis of the breast: a clinicopathologic study of 37 patients with 8.7-year follow-up. Cancer 1996;77(12):2529–2537
3. López-Ferrer P, Jiménez-Heffernan JA, Vicandi B, Ortega L, Viguer JM. Fine needle aspiration cytology of breast fibroadenoma: a cytohistologic correlation study of 405 cases. Acta Cytol 1999;43(4):579–586
4. Tabár L, Dean PB, Tot T. Teaching Atlas of Mammography. 4th ed. Stuttgart/New York: Georg Thieme Verlag; 2012

Chapter 7

Fine-Needle Aspiration or Core Biopsy: A Preoperative Diagnostic Algorithm

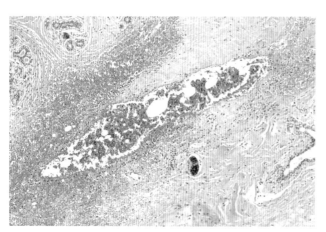

Fig. 7.1

Any procedure involving the use of a needle causes mechanical damage to the targeted tissue. The same is true in cases of fine-needle aspiration or core biopsy of the breast. Necrosis, needle tracks containing blood (**Fig. 7.1**), inflammatory cells, or cholesterol crystals (**Fig. 7.2**) are the most common findings.

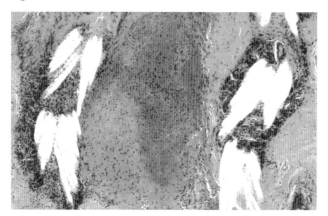

Fig. 7.2

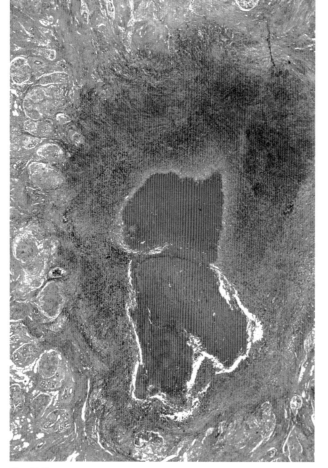

Fig. 7.3

Sometimes an inflammatory pseudotumor forms around the damage (**Fig. 7.3**), with hemosiderin-containing macrophages surrounding the needle tracks (**Fig. 7.4**).

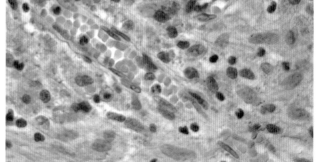

Fig. 7.4

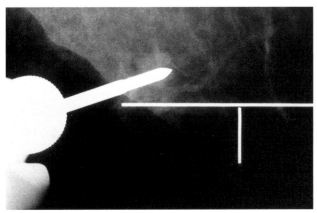

Fig. 7.5

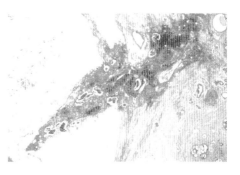

Fig. 7.7

Epithelial displacement may make it difficult for the pathologist to determine the extent of invasion (Figs. 7.6 and 7.7).

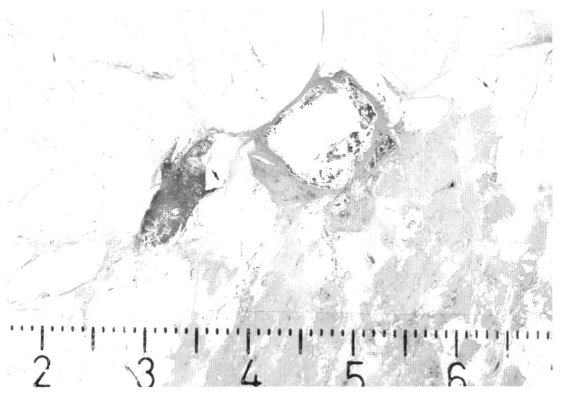

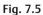

Fig. 7.6

There is insufficient evidence to determine whether or not a needle biopsy procedure (Fig. 7.5) can initiate metastatic tumor spread, but this possibility cannot be ruled out. Because of this uncertainty, we recommend a restrictive approach when using these procedures.

The aim of the diagnostic needle biopsy procedure is to obtain the minimum representative tissue needed for a definite preoperative diagnosis, while at the same time causing least harm to the patient (compare Figs. 7.8 and 7.9).

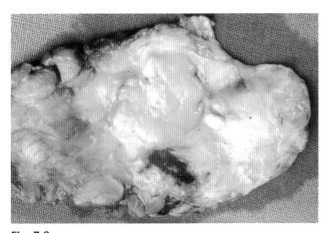

Fig. 7.8

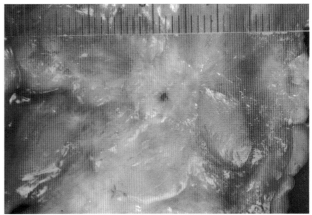

Fig. 7.9

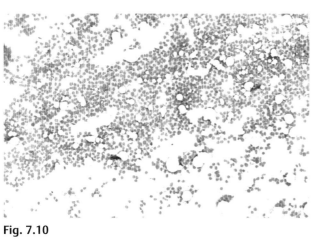

Fig. 7.10

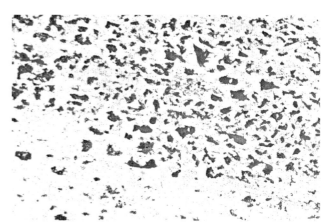

Fig. 7.11

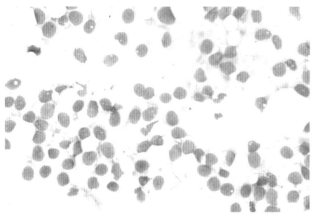

Fig. 7.12

Fine-needle aspiration biopsy (FNAB) is a simple, quick, and very useful method for the preoperative diagnosis of breast lesions. In experienced hands when used in conjunction with clinical and radiological findings, FNAB has high sensitivity, specificity, and accuracy. Core biopsy provides a contiguous cylinder of tissue for histological analysis and is easier to interpret. It is replacing FNAB in many institutions.

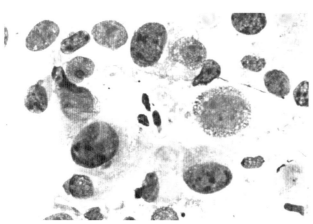

Fig. 7.13

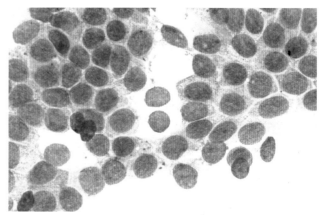

Fig. 7.14

Fig. 7.15

Fig. 7.16

Fig. 7.17

The most useful cytological diagnostic criteria of malignancy are as follows:

- *High cellularity* (compare **Figs. 7.10** and **7.11**)
- *Absence of myoepithelial cells* (seen best in benign lesions as small, oval, bare nuclei, single or in pairs, in the background of the smear [**Fig. 7.12**])
- *Loss of cohesiveness* of the epithelial cells (compare **Figs. 7.13** and **7.14**)
- *Cellular atypia* (compare **Figs. 7.15** and **7.16**).

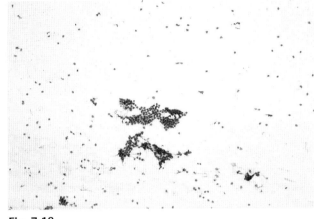

Fig. 7.18

The goals of FNAB are not to rule out but to verify a malignancy, if possible, and to categorize the cytological picture rather than to type and grade the lesions. FNAB categorizes the cytological picture as follows:

II—Unsatisfactory sample (**Fig. 7.17**)

III—Benign, no cytological signs of malignancy (**Fig. 7.18**)

IV—Suspicious for malignancy (**Fig. 7.19**)

V—Malignant (**Fig. 7.20**)

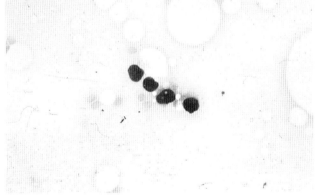

Fig. 7.19

Category I is reserved for cases without preoperative FNAB (see **Fig. 7.23**).

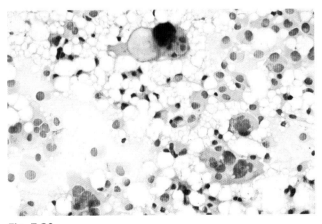

Fig. 7.20

The system presented here is sufficient for correct preoperative categorization of the findings. More detailed and complicated systems of reporting categories for both FNAB and core biopsies have been published and are recommended in different guidelines.

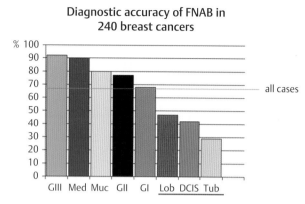

Fig. 7.21

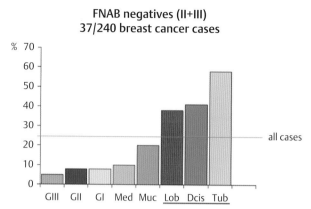

Fig. 7.22

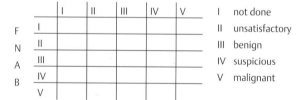

Fig. 7.23

Figs. 7.21 and 7.22 show our data on the accuracy of FNAB according to tumor grade and type. Although grade III carcinomas and medullary and mucinous carcinomas are easy to sample and interpret, the opposite is true for invasive lobular carcinomas, tubular carcinomas, and ductal carcinoma in situ (DCIS). The cytologist has to continuously follow up the results of preoperative FNAB, comparing them with the postoperative histological outcome. A simple method of comparison uses the table shown in **Fig. 7.23**. On the basis of these data, statistical parameters such as sensitivity, specificity, accuracy, and false-negative and false-positive rates can be calculated. An unsatisfactory rate less than 20%, absolute sensitivity over 60%, and complete sensitivity (malignant + suspicious FNABs/malignant outcome) over 80% are the suggested minimum standards. Most importantly, the false-positive rate must be as near to zero as possible.

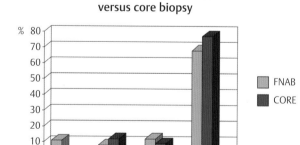

Fig. 7.24

Core biopsy allows definitive preoperative histological diagnoses in most of the representative sample cases (**Figs. 7.25** and **7.26**). This procedure has a slightly higher average accuracy compared with FNAB (**Figs. 7.24** and **7.27**). We found this procedure to be particularly useful in cases of lobular invasive carcinoma, tubular carcinoma, and DCIS (see Chapter 10, Cases 4 and 5).

Another advantage of core biopsy is that benign conditions, especially fibroadenoma, can be easily diagnosed (see Chapter 6).

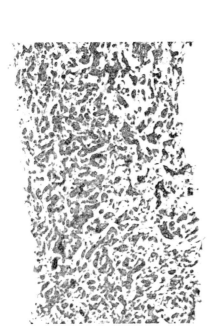

Fig. 7.25

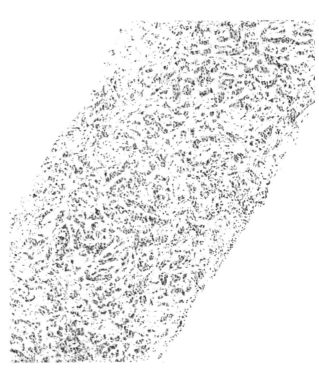

Fig. 7.26

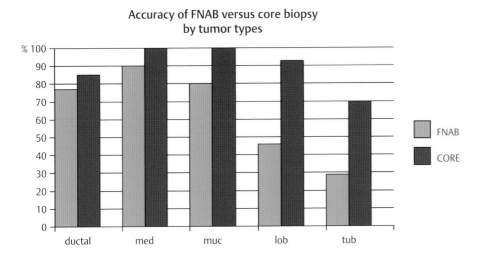

Accuracy of FNAB versus core biopsy by tumor types

Fig. 7.27

Preoperative Diagnostic Algorithm

Following an adequate preoperative workup, most of the surgically removed tumors will have a malignant histologic diagnosis. About 75% of the lesions referred to surgical intervention, benign and malignant combined, will be circular or stellate masses on the mammogram with or without associated microcalcifications. Nearly 25% of the lesions referred to surgery will be microcalcifications on the mammogram without an associated tumor mass. Approximately 3% of the cases will be operated on after galactography.

A. *Round/Oval-Shaped* Radiopaque Densities on the Mammogram (**Fig. 7.28**)

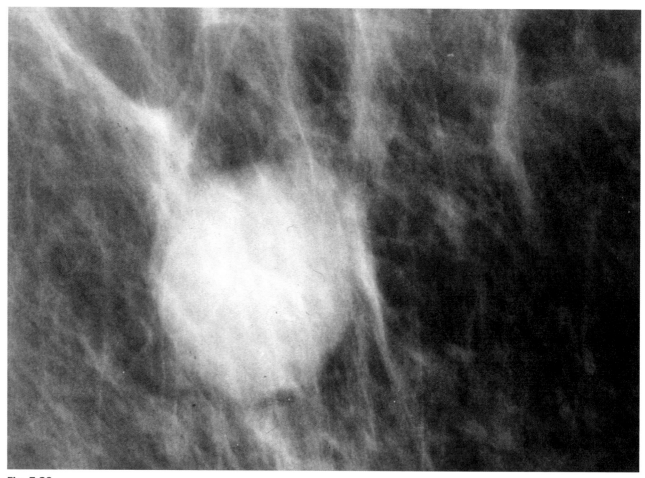

Fig. 7.28

Only about 60% of the surgically removed circular or oval lesions will be malignant at histologic examination. The remainder consists of fibroadenomas, fibrocystic change, and papillomas. Most of the cysts could be treated by aspiration, and they are not included in the percentage of the benign operated circular lesions.

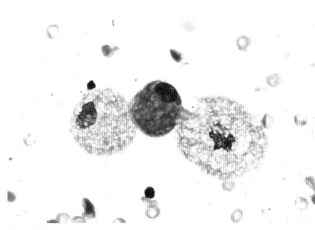

Fig. 7.29

A1—Round/oval radiopaque densities, cystic at ultrasound examination.

A1a—When breast ultrasound examination shows a simple cyst without intracystic growth, cyst aspiration depends on the clinical setting and patient concerns. Cytological examination of the fluid removed from a simple cyst is not necessary. The cytological image otherwise shows low cellularity, foam cells, and apocrine cells (**Figs. 7.29** and **7.30**).

A1b—When breast ultrasound shows intracystic growth, fine-needle aspiration and core biopsy are unreliable methods and may cause pseudoinvasion. Open surgical biopsy and histological examination of the lesion and the surrounding tissue are necessary to arrive at a definite diagnosis (see Chapter 6). Intracystic papillary tumor may be suspected based on large papillary cell groups in the aspirated fluid (**Figs. 7.31** and **7.32**).

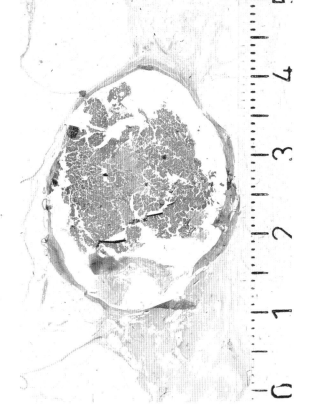

Fig. 7.30

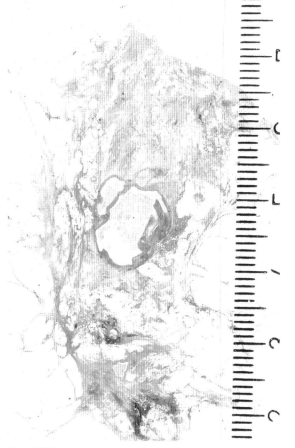

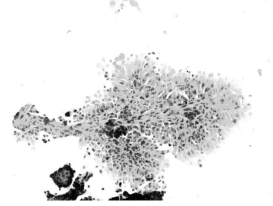

Fig. 7.31

Fig. 7.32

A2—Round/oval radiopaque densities on the mammogram, *solid* on ultrasound.

A2a—Clinically and/or mammographically malignant round/oval radiopaque lesion that is solid at ultrasound examination requires fine-needle aspiration or core biopsy.

If the cytologic diagnosis is malignant, the diagnosis is definite.

If the cytologic diagnosis is suspicious for malignancy core biopsy should be performed.

If the cytologic diagnosis is benign, core biopsy should be performed.

If the aspirated material is inadequate for cytologic examination, then core biopsy should be performed.

In addition to establishing the malignant diagnosis, core biopsy gives information about the in situ or invasive character of the cancer, but in a small proportion of the cases, only the in situ component of otherwise invasive carcinoma is represented in the cores.

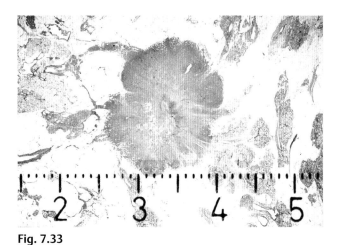

Fig. 7.33

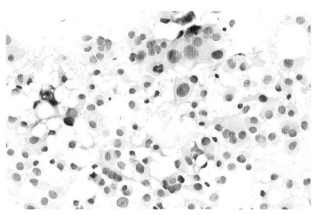

Fig. 7.34

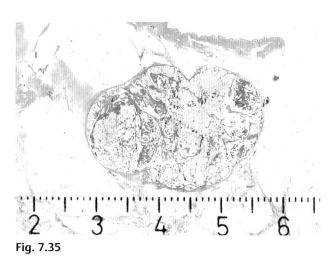

Fig. 7.35

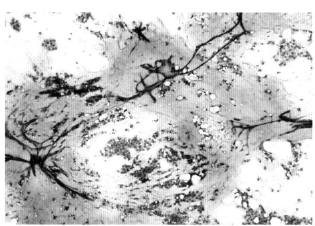

Fig. 7.36

A2b—If the lesion is benign at clinical, mammographic and ultrasound examination: core biopsy should be performed.

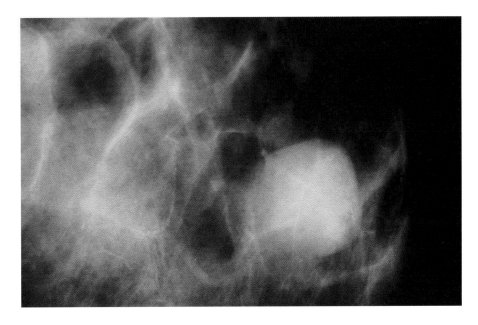

Fig. 7.37

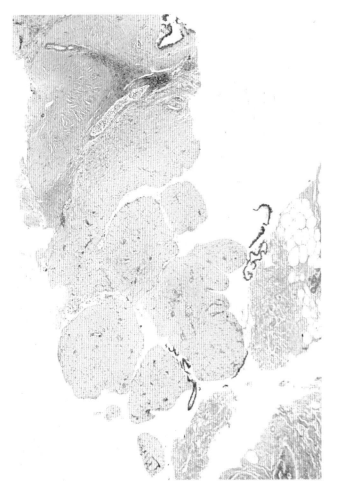

Fig. 7.38

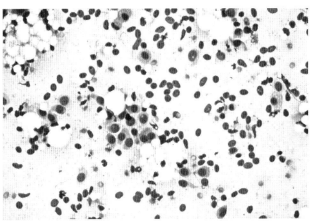

Fig. 7.39

Comment

The malignant round or oval lesions will most often be invasive ductal NST carcinomas grade II or III (**Figs. 7.33** and **7.34**), medullary or mucinous carcinomas. They can be diagnosed easily by fine-needle aspiration because of their cellularity, obvious cellular atypia, and, in the case of mucinous carcinoma, by the presence of mucin (**Figs. 7.35** and **7.36**). The most commonly encountered benign circular solid lesion is a fibroadenoma (**Fig. 7.37**). It is easily diagnosed on core biopsy (**Fig. 7.38**), but cytology often provides a cellular picture with moderate atypia (**Fig. 7.39**); this is the most common source of a false-positive FNAB diagnosis.

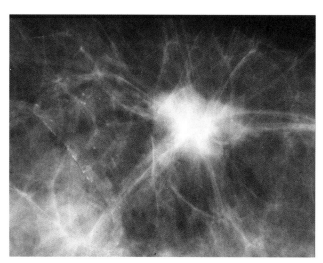

Fig. 7.40

B. *Stellate Lesions* on the Mammogram

The stellate lesions on the mammogram will have a malignant histologic diagnosis in 94% of cases.

B1—"*A white star*" on the mammogram (**Fig. 7.40**) requires percutaneous needle biopsy.

If the cytologic diagnosis is malignant the diagnosis is definite. Core biopsy adds information about the invasive nature, histological grade, and type of the lesion.

If the cytologic diagnosis is suspicious for malignancy, core biopsy should be performed.

If the cytologic diagnosis is benign, core biopsy should be performed.

If the aspirated material is inadequate for cytologic examination, then core biopsy should be performed.

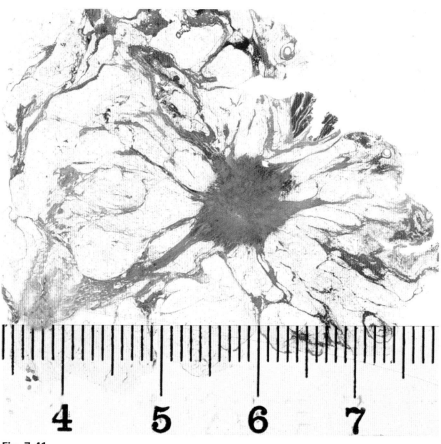

Fig. 7.41

Comment

"White stars" on the mammogram are nearly always malignant, most often ductal NST carcinomas grades I (**Fig. 7.41**) and II, tubular or tubulolobular carcinomas. Stromal desmoplasia may make it difficult to obtain representative cytological material by fine-needle aspiration. Satisfactory cellularity cannot be expected even if the aspiration is repeated. The rare posttraumatic or postoperative stellate scar tissue (**Fig. 7.44**) may cause differential diagnostic difficulties.

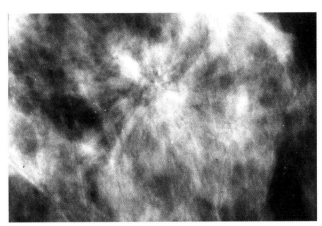

Fig. 7.42

B2—When a *"black star"* is detected on the mammogram, open surgical biopsy is recommended (**Fig. 7.42**).

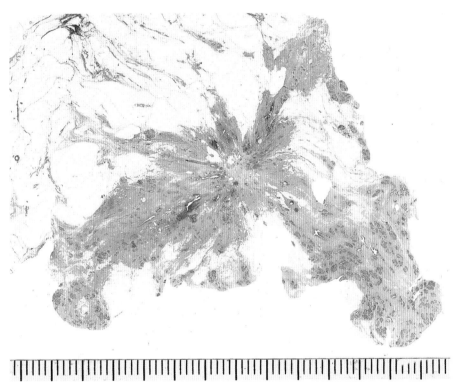

Fig. 7.43

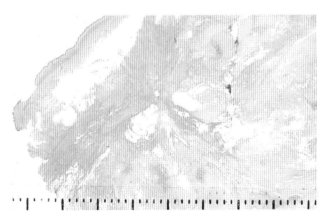

Fig. 7.44

Comment

The black stars on the mammogram correspond to radial scars (**Fig. 7.43**), which may contain foci of ductal hyperplasia, atypical ductal hyperplasia (ADH), atypical lobular hyperplasia (ALH), lobular carcinoma in situ (LCIS), or DCIS grade I in the peripheral areas of the radiating structure ("crown"). In the fibroelastic center, pseudoinfiltrative tubular structures may be present, simulating tubular cancer (see Chapter 6). Cytology is not the method of choice for making the diagnosis of these low-grade lesions. Even core biopsy may provide insufficient material for the differential diagnosis of the aforementioned lesions. The method of choice is large-section histology of the entire lesion.

C. *Microcalcifications* on the Mammogram

C1—When *"casting type"* calcifications are detected on the mammogram (**Fig. 7.45**) (96% probability of malignancy), fine-needle aspiration biopsy, core biopsy, vacuum-assisted or radiofrequency-directed biopsy should be performed.

C2—When *"broken needle–like"* calcifications are detected on the mammogram, (**Fig. 7.46**) (60% probability of malignancy), core biopsy, vacuum-assisted or radiofrequency-directed biopsy should be performed.

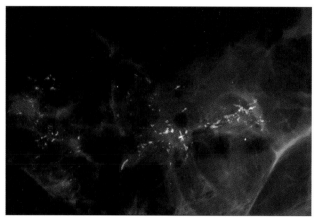

Fig. 7.45

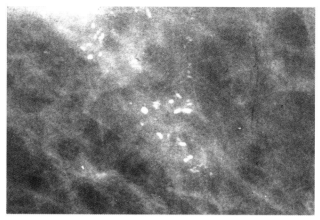

Fig. 7.46

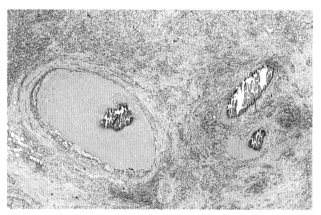

Fig. 7.47

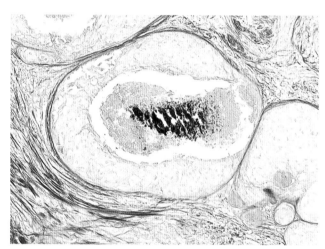

Fig. 7.48

Comment

These calcifications almost always represent DCIS grade III (or II) with or without invasion (**Fig. 7.47**). A definite preoperative morphological diagnosis of malignancy can often be made with cytology because the tumor cells are highly atypical. If it is necessary to prove the presence of invasion preoperatively, core biopsy is required, but its relatively low sensitivity for small foci of invasion must be kept in mind. Vacuum-assisted large bore-needle or radiofrequency-directed biopsies provide more tissue for analysis. Surgical intervention is always necessary.

Comment

These microcalcifications often indicate DCIS grade II, involving an enlarged lobule (**Fig. 7.48**). Differential diagnosis includes papillomas, fibroadenomas, and cases of fibrocystic change (see also comment under C1 about invasion and Chapter 4).

C3—When "*powdery*" microcalcifications are detected on the mammograms (**Fig. 7.49**) (45% probability of malignancy), wide surgical biopsy should be performed.

Novel biopsy techniques provide more tissue for preoperative assessment. Vacuum-assisted large bore-needle biopsy specimens (**Fig. 7.51**) are advantageous for diagnosing DCIS grade III (**Fig. 7.51a**), DCIS grade II and DCIS grade I (**Fig. 7.51b** and **c**). Even larger contiguous tissue is provided when using radiofrequency directed biopsy (**Fig. 7.52**).

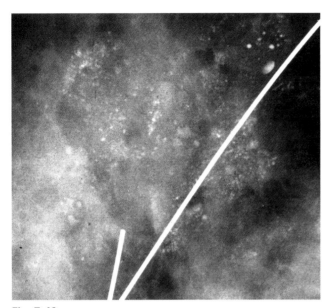

Fig. 7.49

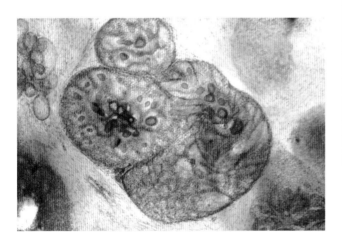

Fig. 7.50

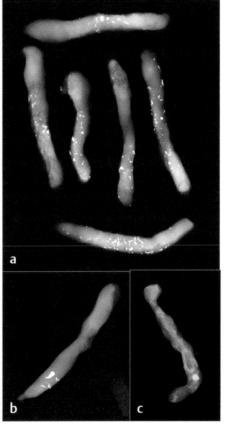

Fig. 7.51a-c

Comment

This mammographic picture indicates the presence of a large number of psammoma body–like microcalcifications in the lumina of the altered TDLUs. This can usually be observed in different types of adenosis, mainly sclerosing adenosis and apocrine metaplasia, but even in DCIS grade I (**Fig. 7.50**, thick-section image). Fine-needle aspiration is inadequate for assessing this grade of DCIS because the cells are highly differentiated. The microcalcifications may be localized in benign structures adjacent to the DCIS and not in the DCIS itself, so that a mammographically directed core biopsy may give a false-negative result.

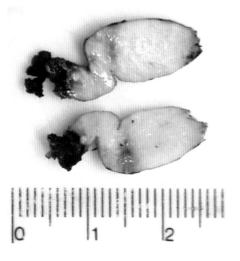

Fig. 7.52

Although the described preoperative diagnostic algorithm is useful for characterizing the individual radiologically detected lesions, the preoperative interdisciplinary diagnosis should represent a summation of all available clinical, radiological, and morphological information regarding the case. This is best achieved if the cases are discussed at a tumor board in the presence of breast radiologists, surgeons, oncologists, and pathologists.

The aim of the preoperative diagnosis is to achieve proper therapeutic decisions. Choosing the type of surgical intervention requires adequate assessment of the size of the lesion, distribution of the lesions (unifocal, multifocal, or diffuse), and, especially, the extent of the disease (see Chapter 2). The location of the lesion(s) within the breast (distance to pectoralis muscle, skin, or nipple) is also important. In preoperative settings, these parameters can only be provided by the radiologist. The decision about preoperative neoadjuvant therapy is also based on radiological and clinical staging of the disease.

Multimodality breast radiology (combining mammography, ultrasound examination, magnetic resonance imaging, and other imaging modalities) is highly accurate in determining the tumor size and categorizing cases as early (**Fig. 7.53**) or advanced (**Fig. 7.54**). It is also able to rule out or prove multifocality (**Figs. 7.55** and **7.56**) or diffuse distribution of the lesions (**Fig. 7.57**) and to delineate extensive multifocal or diffuse tumors from those having limited extent (**Figs. 7.55** and **7.56**) with high accuracy. Taking needle biopsies from the most distant foci of a cancer increases this accuracy to nearly 100%, making interdisciplinary preoperative diagnosis of breast lesions the gold standard. Noncalcified (usually grade I or II) DCIS, LCIS, small (< 5 mm) invasive tumor foci and rare cases of invasive lobular carcinoma may remain radiologically undetected, even in the multimodality imaging era, and lead to discrepancies in radiological–pathological correlation.

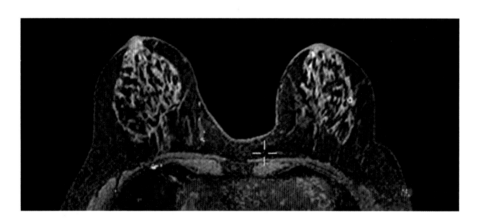

Fig. 7.53

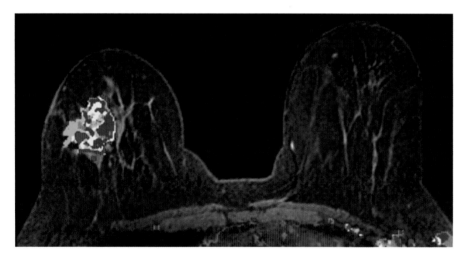

Fig. 7.54

Breast radiology provides important prognostic information in many cases. Early (< 15 mm) stellate lesions and powdery microcalcifications indicate excellent prognosis; large, rapidly growing spherical/oval masses, extensive architectural distortion, and the presence of casting-type microcalcifications are all negative prognostic parameters.

Estrogen and progesterone receptors, c-erb-B2 expression, and proliferative activity of the tumor cells can be adequately assessed on preoperative biopsy and guide the preoperative oncological therapy, if needed. Quantification of the receptors is more accurate on core biopsy than on FNAB.

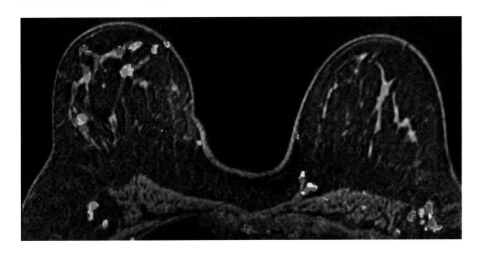

Fig. 7.55

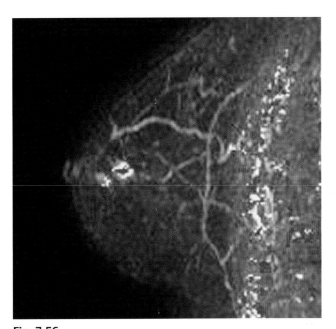

Fig. 7.56

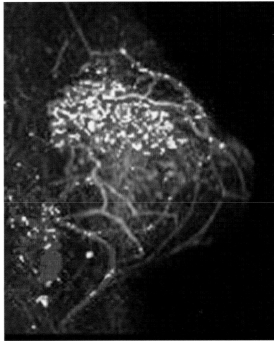

Fig. 7.57

Conclusions

This preoperative diagnostic algorithm represents a synthesis of the accumulated knowledge about the clinical, radiological, and morphological characteristics of breast diseases and the accumulated experience about the advantages and disadvantages of biopsy techniques. It also represents a rational method for using preoperative diagnostic procedures such as fine-needle aspiration biopsy, core biopsy, large bore-needle biopsies, and surgical excisional biopsy. The preoperative diagnostic procedure has to be as harmless as possible for the patient and cause as few as possible changes to the tumor. Fibroadenomas and papillomas may yield cellular and atypical aspirates, which in turn may lead to a false-positive cytological diagnosis. Core biopsy has a better ability to prove the benign nature of the lesions than fine-needle aspiration biopsy. On the other hand, ruling out malignancy is sometimes, especially in low-grade lesions, impossible by FNAB or core biopsy. In these cases, wide surgical excision is indicated. Most importantly, the pathologists must correlate their findings with radiological findings and understand the clinical relevance of all the details in the pathological report.

Bibliography

1. Willis SL, Ramzy I. Analysis of false results in a series of 835 fine needle aspirates of breast lesions. Acta Cytol 1995;39(5):858–864
2. Tot T, Tabár L, Gere M. The role of core needle biopsy of breast lesions when fine needle aspiration biopsy is inconclusive (Summary). Acta Cytologica 1999;43:707
3. Tabár L, Dean PB, Kaufman CS, Duffy SW, Chen HH. A new era in the diagnosis of breast cancer. Surg Oncol Clin N Am 2000;9(2):233–277
4. Perry N, Puthaar E; *European Commission. Directorate-General for Health and Consumer Protection,* et al. European Guidelines for Quality Assurance in Breast Cancer Screening and Diagnosis. 4th ed. Luxembourg, Belgium; Office for Official Publications of the European Communities; 2006:222–248
5. Tot T, Gere M. Radiological-pathological correlation in diagnosing breast carcinoma: the role of pathology in the multimodality era. Pathol Oncol Res 2008;14(2):173–178
6. Tot T, Tabár L. The role of radiological-pathological correlation in diagnosing early breast cancer: the pathologist's perspective. Virchows Arch 2011;458(2):125–131

Chapter 8

The Postoperative Workup

To determine the real extent, size, and distribution of the lesions in the excised breast tissue, the histological findings need to be directly correlated with the clinical, radiological, and macroscopic findings. To accomplish this correlation, the pathologist should prepare and examine sections of tissue that are as large and as continuous as possible. To this end,

the technique of large histological sections is unquestionably superior to the traditional small-block technique.

The production of a two-dimensional large-section image needs to be carefully planned. The method of the cut-up of the specimen differs according to the type of the operation (mastectomy or segmentectomy/quadrantectomy) and lesion (microcalcifications, solitary, or multiple tumors).

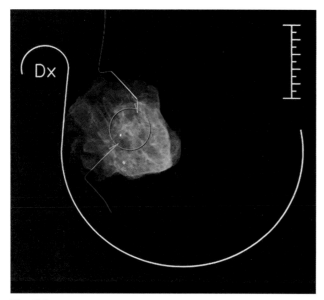

Fig. 8.1

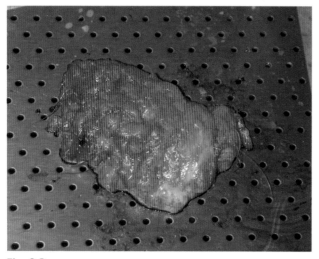

Fig. 8.2

The specimen is received in a fresh state after specimen radiography is performed to confirm the presence of the preoperatively diagnosed radiological abnormality within it. The specimen radiograph (Fig. 8.1) assists the pathologist in planning the cut-up to include a cross section of the entire abnormality in a single large section. Accessories such as the EasyMarkSpecimen device (Medicinsk Innovations Design MID AB, Stockholm, Sweden) facilitate documenting the position of the lesion and orientation of the specimen. Thorough macroscopic examination of the specimen is also important. The size of the specimen should be measured in three dimensions, and the number and type of the marking sutures (Figs. 8.2 and 8.3) and the number and position of the guide wires should be recorded. Because the specimen consists of soft breast tissue atop a firm base (radiographic film, table), it usually takes the form of a relatively flat piece of tissue (Figs. 8.2 and 8.3). The larger tumors are firmer and are usually easily located by inspection and palpation. The smaller tumors are not directly seen on macroscopic examination of the unsliced specimen but are often palpable and are usually easily seen on the specimen radiograph. If the specimen contains only radiologically detected microcalcifications or a small nonpalpable tumor, finding the appropriate plane for slicing is totally dependent upon careful mammographic guidance. In the latter situation, it is best to slice the specimen horizontally (parallel with the table) in the plane of the specimen radiograph (Figs. 8.4 and 8.5). This is recommended even in the presence of a solitary well-defined tumor mass. Multiple tumors are more difficult to demonstrate in a single large section. In these cases, the plane for slicing should be chosen based on palpation of the entire specimen and on evaluation of the specimen radiograph. Correlation with the findings on magnetic resonance imaging is also very helpful.

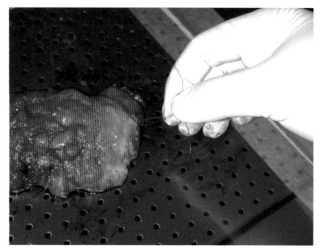

Fig. 8.3

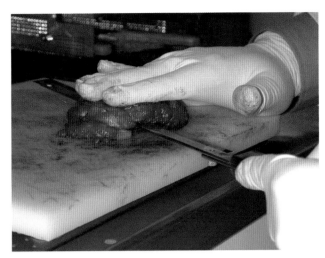

Fig. 8.4

A knife with a very sharp disposable blade is needed for slicing a fresh breast specimen. The blade must be changed after every two or three breast specimens are cut, more often when very hard or calcified tissue is encountered. It is more dangerous for the pathologist to use a dull blade than to use a very sharp one. Inexperienced pathologists are advised to use a translucent plastic plate to push the specimen against the table instead of holding it directly with their hand (**Fig. 8.6**).

The slices should be 3- to 4-mm thick (**Figs. 8.7** and **8.8**). A considerable variation in thickness within the same slice or among slices can markedly reduce the technical quality of the specimen mammograms and histological sections. The slices need to be thoroughly examined macroscopically. The well-formed tumor masses should be described and measured in millimeters. The relation of the tumors to the resection margins must be described in terms of the minimum number of millimeters of tumor-free margins. A lengthy macroscopic description is unnecessary because the cut surface of the entire specimen is demonstrated on the large histological sections.

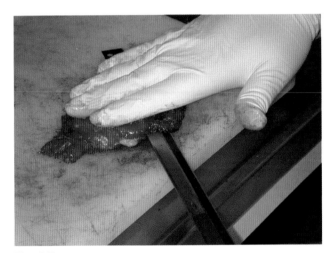

Fig. 8.5

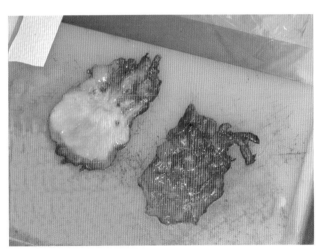

Fig. 8.7

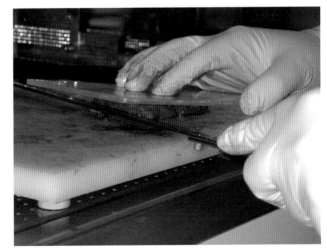

Fig. 8.6

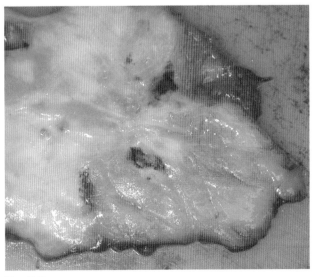

Fig. 8.8

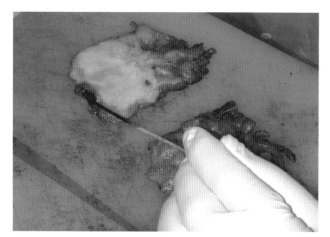

Fig. 8.9

With this technique it is not necessary to ink the surface of the specimen, but colored inks should be used to mark the position of the marking sutures (**Fig. 8.9**).

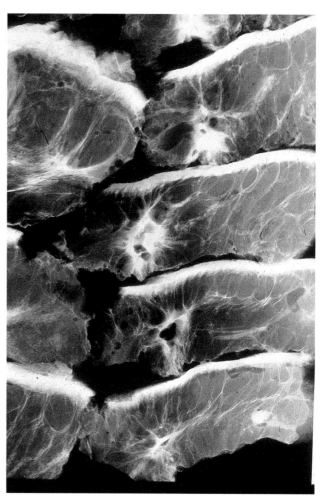

Fig. 8.10

The 3- to 4-mm slices then undergo repeat specimen radiography. The radiographic examination of the slices (**Fig. 8.10**) is always a useful procedure and is absolutely necessary in cases with mammographically detected microcalcifications, those with multifocal tumors, and those with nonpalpable lesions. The radiologist compares the mammographic findings and the findings on specimen radiography with the radiological images of the macroslices, and then marks the slices that have radiological abnormalities. The pathologist must correlate the macroscopic findings in the marked slices with the radiological abnormalities. The most representative slices are selected for embedding and processing: the slices with the largest tumor diameter, those containing the largest number of tumor foci in the cases with multifocal tumors, those containing macroscopically and/or radiologically discernible nonmalignant lesions, and those containing microcalcifications. It is worth mentioning that pathologists are fully responsible for tissue sampling, even with radiological assistance. Therefore, they are encouraged to sample all suspicious macroscopic abnormalities, even those that have not been marked by the radiologist.

The recommended average number of selected slices per case is two to four. At this step, small tissue blocks may be taken for immunohistochemistry, image analysis, flow cytometry, and molecular biological examinations, and/or tissue banking, but the most representative slices must be left intact. Because the reliability of the histological diagnosis of mammographically detected and macroscopically poorly defined lesions depends upon mammographic–pathological correlation, one adequate large section is more important than the additional examinations. In these cases, especially if the lesion is smaller than 10 mm in the largest dimension, sampling of the tumor tissue for special examinations or taking intraoperative frozen sections is contraindicated.

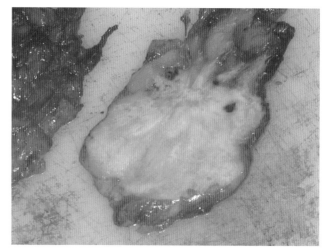

Fig. 8.11

Large histological sections provide an ideal tool for assessing the circumferential resection margins (Fig. 8.11). The superficial and the deep resection margins are not directly demonstrated because the specimen is sectioned horizontally. Absence of radiological and macroscopic abnormalities in the first and the last horizontally taken slice provides indirect proof that the margins are free of tumor along both these surfaces. Should one or both of these slices contain a tumor or other abnormality, it is necessary to complete the sampling of the tissue by small tissue blocks that demonstrate the margins over and under the tumor (Fig. 8.12).

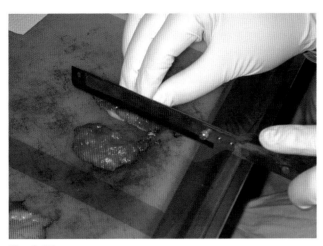

Fig. 8.12

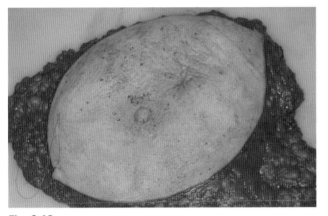

Fig. 8.13

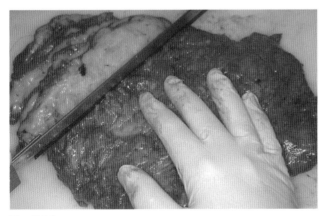

Fig. 8.14

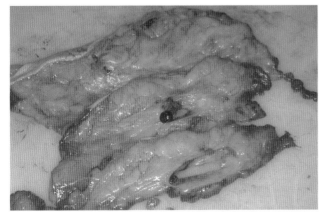

Fig. 8.15

Slicing the mastectomy specimen (Fig. 8.13) for large-section histology is a different procedure for two practical reasons: the cut surface of the specimen is usually much larger than the dimensions of the routinely used large-section glasses and, more importantly, the posterior resection margin (and not the circumferential as in segmentectomy) is the only important one in the case of mastectomy. Therefore, the large section must demonstrate the posterior surgical margin. The specimen is sliced sagittally (in a plane perpendicular to the resection margin of the mastectomy specimen) (Figs. 8.14 and 8.15). Parallel slices 3- to 4-mm thick are produced and analyzed precisely in the manner previously described. One must keep in mind that the radiograph of the mastectomy specimen is taken with the nipple "en face" but the radiographs of the slices are taken with the nipple in profile. The specimen slice radiographs need to be correlated with both the mediolateral and the craniocaudal mammographic projection images. Whereas the breasts are compressed during mammographic examination, they are freely hanging during magnetic resonance imaging. This influences the position of the lesions within the breast and the dimensions of the diseased area, which has to be taken into account when correlating radiological and histological findings.

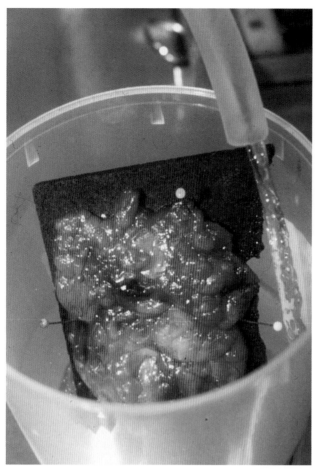

Fig. 8.16

Tissue Processing

The selected tissue slices are stretched on a cork plate and pinned, with the surface to be cut with the microtome facing down. The slices are immersed in dishes containing standard formalin solution for tissue fixation (**Fig. 8.16**). By fixing the tissue when it is stretched, a fairly flat surface can be achieved. The slices are then fixed for 24 hours. Thorough fixation of the slices is essential; suboptimal fixation causes difficulties on sectioning. Microwave treatment can considerably diminish the time necessary for optimal fixation, but routines must be developed in every laboratory that introduces this more rapid technique. After fixation, the slices are removed from the cork plate and placed into a sufficiently large container within an automatic tissue processor. Before processing, slices that are already fixed can be trimmed to get the ideal thickness of 3 to 4 mm throughout the whole slice.

Sectioning of the large blocks (**Figs. 8.17, 8.18,** and **8.19**) is performed using a special microtome. The most important factor in obtaining large histological sections of proper quality is the skillful and experienced technician.

Staining is performed using modified holders, which are placed in the same automatic stainer used for small blocks. The recipe for hematoxylin and eosin staining is the same as for small blocks. The large section produced this way has the same staining quality as the conventional small histology slides (**Fig. 8.20**).

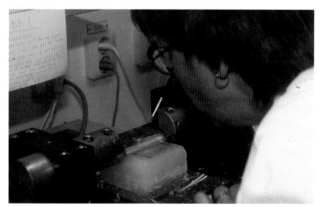

Fig. 8.17

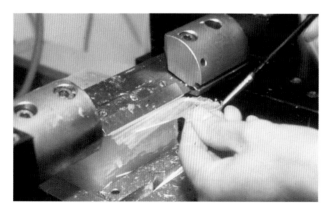

Fig. 8.18

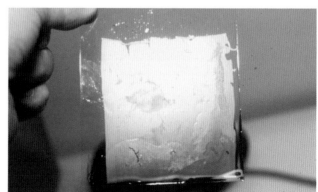

Fig. 8.19

Summary of the Steps of Macroscopic Examination

I. Nonmastectomy Specimen

1. Studying the radiograph of the intact surgical specimen
2. Inspecting and describing the whole specimen
3. Measuring the whole specimen
4. Palpating the specimen
5. Slicing the specimen into slices 3- to 4-mm thick, parallel with the table
6. Placing the slices sequentially on plastic films
7. Macroscopically examining the cut surfaces of the slices
8. Measuring the largest tumor dimensions
9. Sampling or aspirating material for tissue banking, receptor analysis, or research purposes
10. Marking the suture position with ink
11. Covering the slices with film and marking them with numbers
12. Obtaining specimen radiographs of the slices with and without microfocus magnification
13. Comparing the radiological and macroscopic abnormalities
14. Selecting the most representative slices
15. Sampling small blocks for additional methods (in macroscopically detectable lesions larger than 10 mm)

II. Mastectomy Specimen

1–4. Same as for a nonmastectomy specimen
5. Slicing the specimen sagittally, perpendicular to the table
6–15. Same as for a nonmastectomy specimen

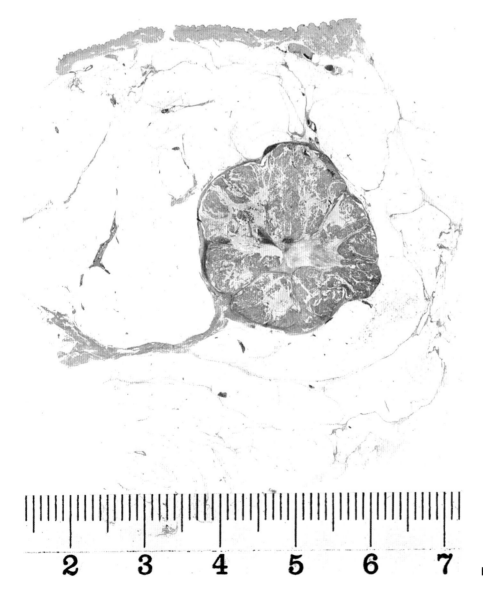

Fig. 8.20

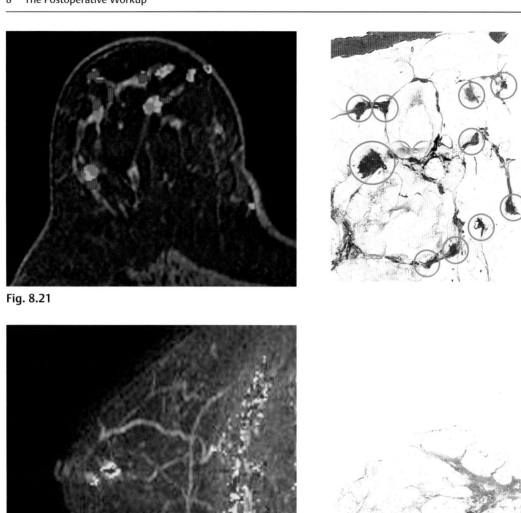

Fig. 8.21

Fig. 8.22

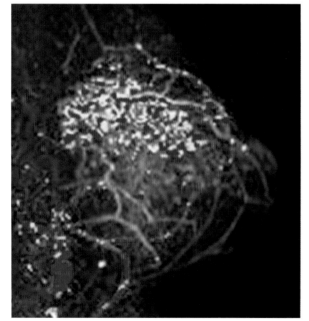

Fig. 8.23

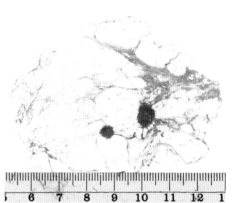

Fig. 8.24

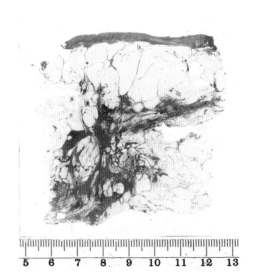

Fig. 8.25

Fig. 8.26

The microscopic analysis of large histological sections should begin with determining the disease extent. Approaching from the periphery of the section, the pathologist should mark the most peripheral malignant structures (in situ or invasive) and repeat the process from all directions. The result will be a marked area representing a cross section through the diseased tissue. The space the malignant structures occupy in the breast rarely shows the regular shape of a geometric body; it is almost always irregular. This means that the extent of the disease varies at different levels of the specimen and in different projections. Consequently, it is often necessary to summarize the findings in adjacent tissue slices and/or tissue slices taken at different levels of the specimen to determine the real extent of the disease. The next step is determining the distribution of the lesions within the marked area. By finding and marking well-delineated foci of invasive and in situ carcinoma, the pathologist documents multifocality (**Figs. 8.21, 8.22, 8.23, and 8.24**). Such well-delineated foci are not found in diffuse lesions (**Figs. 8.25 and 8.26**). Unifocal lesion are characterized with a single well-delineated focus that is equal to or slightly smaller (in case of the presence of a peritumoral in situ component) than the extent (**Fig. 8.28**).

By finding and measuring the largest invasive focus, the pathologist assesses the size of the tumor. By measuring the distance between the nearest malignant structures and the resection margins the pathologist determines the completeness of the surgical intervention. Radiological–pathological correlation is essential in determining all these parameters.

The realistic aim of radiological–pathological correlation is to properly categorize the cases as extensive (≥ 40 mm extent) (**Figs. 8.21** and **8.22**) or of limited extent (**Figs. 8.23** and **8.24**), and as early (< 15 mm invasive tumor size) (**Figs. 8.27** and **8.28**) or more advanced (**Figs. 8.29** and **8.30**), rather than aiming to achieve a millimetric concordance. In the multimodality imaging era, over 80% of cases are properly categorized by radiologists. As mentioned previously, in addition to technical factors, discrepancies are often related to the presence of noncalcified low-grade in situ tumor components and very small invasive tumor foci that are not visible with radiological examinations.

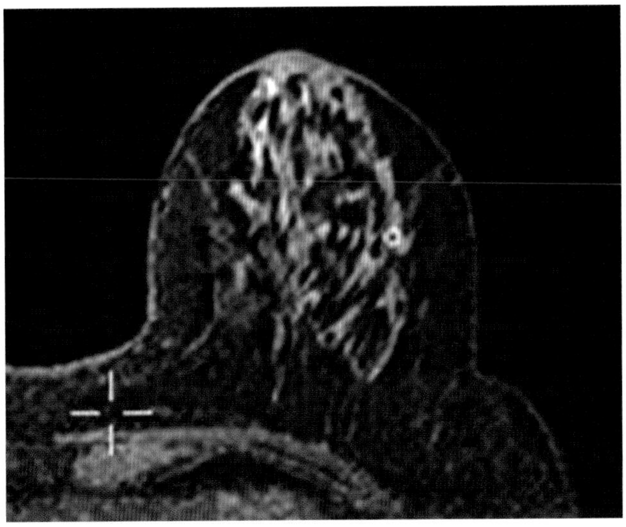

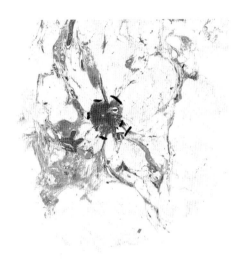

Fig. 8.28

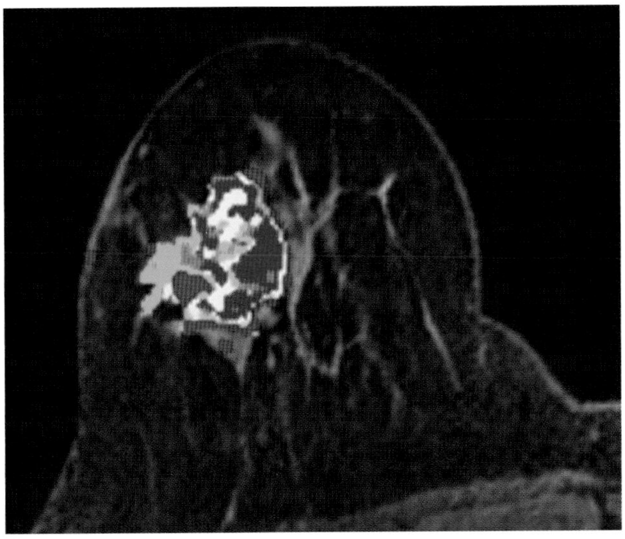

Fig. 8.27

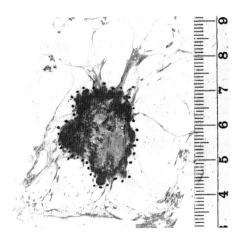

Fig. 8.30

Fig. 8.29

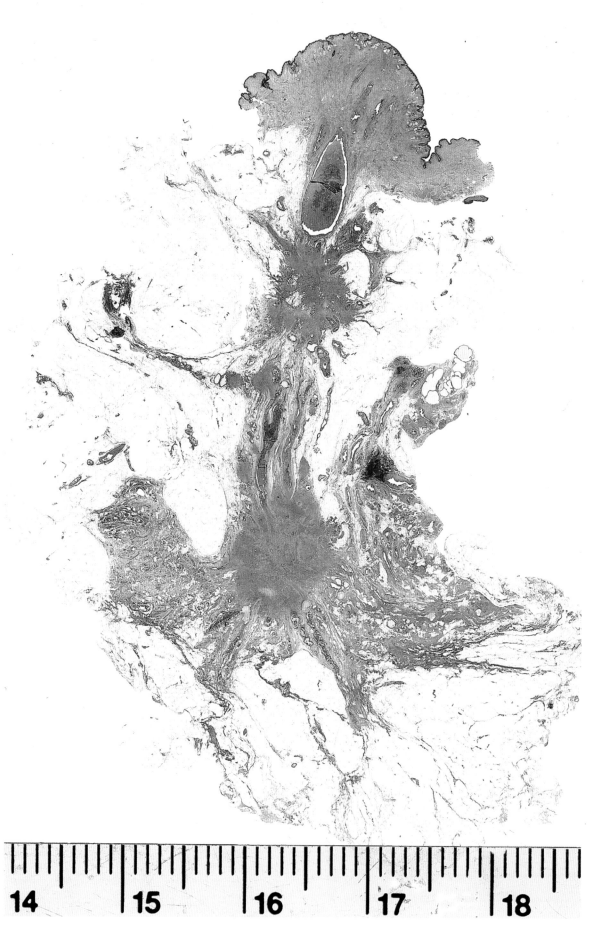

Fig. 8.31

Advantages of the Large-Section Technique

1. Demonstrates the entire lesion in one or several cross sections, which allows for the following:
   - ❏ Documentation of the tumor size
   - ❏ Assessment of the intratumoral heterogeneity
   - ❏ Assessment of the effects of diagnostic and/or therapeutic procedures

2. Demonstrates the tumor together with its environment, enabling the following:
   - ❏ Documentation of the multifocal/multicentric nature of the tumor
   - ❏ Assessment of the in situ components within and surrounding the tumor
   - ❏ Assessment of the tumor's relationship to surrounding benign changes and normal tissue

3. Demonstrates a large area of the resection margins for the following:
   - ❏ Direct assessment of the completeness (radicality) of the excision
   - ❏ Direct measurement of the distance of the tumor from the margin
   - ❏ Direct demonstration of malignant or premalignant changes at the margin

4. Allows a direct correlation of the histological findings with the radiologically suspicious findings

Conclusions

Large histological sections accurately demonstrate the size of the tumor, the extent of the disease, the distribution of the in situ and invasive components of the carcinoma, the presence or absence of intratumoral and intertumoral heterogeneity, and the surgical margin in one plane (**Fig. 8.31**). This technique is cost-effective, simple, and represents a prerequisite for successful radiological–pathological correlation.

Bibliography

1. Jackson PA, Merchant W, McCormick CJ, Cook MG. A comparison of large block macrosectioning and conventional techniques in breast pathology. Virchows Arch 1994;425(3):243–248
2. Foschini MP, Tot T, Eusebi V. Large-section (macrosection) histologic slides. In: Silverstein MJ, ed. Ductal Carcinoma In Situ of the Breast. 2nd ed. Philadelphia, PA: Lippincott; 2002:249–254
3. Tabár L, Tot T, Dean PB. Breast Cancer: The Art and Science of Early Detection with Mammography. New York, NY: Thieme; 2005:405–438
4. Tot T. The subgross morphology of the normal and pathologically altered breast tissue. In: Suri J, Rangayyan R, eds. Recent Advances in Breast Imaging, Mammography, and Computer-Aided Diagnosis of Breast Cancer. Bellingham, WA: SPIE Press; 2006:1–49
5. Tot T. Cost-benefit analysis of using large-format histology sections in routine diagnostic breast care. Breast 2010;19(4):284–288
6. Tot T. Large-format histology, a prerequisite for adequate assessment of early breast carcinomas. In: Kahán ZS, Tot T, eds. Breast Cancer: A Heterogeneous Disease Entity. New York, NY: Springer; 2011:57–88
7. Tot T, Eusebi V, Ibarra JA (Guest editors). Large section histology in diagnosing breast carcinoma. Int J Breast Cancer special issue, 2012, open access publication

Chapter 9

Assessment of the Most Important Prognostic Parameters

In addition to clinical prognostic factors (e.g., patient age or socioeconomic status), genetic factors (e.g., presence of BRCA1 or BRCA2 mutation), radiological factors (e.g., casting type calcifications), there are several morphological parameters that are used in predicting the outcome of the disease. The radiological/surgical morphological prognostic parameters (tumor size, disease extent, lesion distribution, surgical margins, location of the tumor within the breast, and axillary lymph node status) are decisive in choosing adequate surgical intervention but are also associated with disease-specific and/or disease-free survival of the patients. The oncological morphological prognostic parameters (presence or absence of distant metastasis, lymph node status, tumor size, histology grade, receptor status, proliferative activity, and molecular phenotype of the tumor) are decisive in choosing adequate oncological therapy and are related to survival, and some of them are also used to predict the patients' response to the applied therapy (predictive parameters).

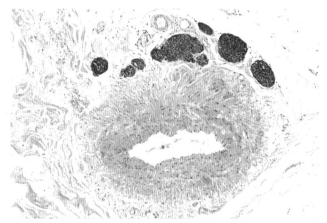

Fig. 9.1

Peritumoral or intratumoral *vascular invasion* (**Fig. 9.1**) is the first step in spreading the tumor cells. These tumor cells may remain within the breast and form secondary invasive foci ("secondary type" of tumor multifocality) or leave the breast via the lymph or blood vessels.

Via the bloodstream the cancer cells (or cancer stem cells) can reach distant organs in which they can survive in dormancy or develop metastatic tumor foci. The presence of *distant metastasis* is the most powerful prognostic factor (**Figs. 9.2** and **9.3**).

Most of the lymph from the breast is first transported toward the subareolar Sappey plexus and then to the axilla through the sentinel nodes. As the first target of lymphatic tumor spread, the sentinel nodes are indicative of the axillary lymph node status. Some lymph vessels from the medial half of the breast lead the lymph to the internal mammary lymph nodes.

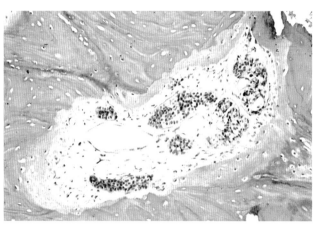

Fig. 9.2

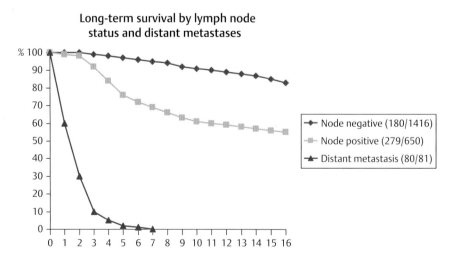

Fig. 9.3 (Based on data of the Swedish Two County study. Women, 40–74 years, were included.)

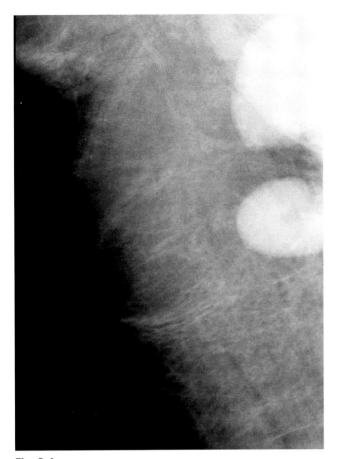

Fig. 9.4

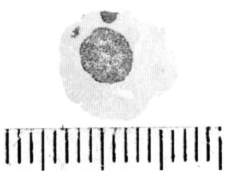

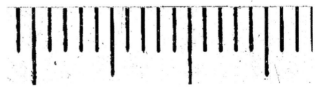

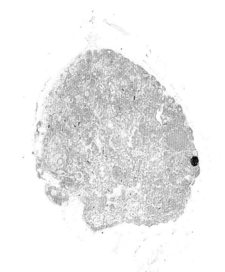

Fig. 9.5

Fig. 9.6

As shown in **Fig. 9.3**, the presence of metastasis in axillary lymph nodes is also a powerful prognostic factor and is important for therapeutic decision-making. This is particularly true if the size of the metastatic deposit(s) is larger than 2.0 mm (so-called macrometastasis, **Figs. 9.4** and **9.5**). Periglandular infiltration and the presence of more than three involved nodes are additional negative prognostic factors. The clinical importance of *micrometastases* (> 0.2 mm but not > 2.0 mm, **Fig. 9.6**) is still debated in the literature. The cancer cells may be individually dispersed in the lymph node and not form a cohesive deposit (**Fig. 9.7**). In such cases 200 tumor cells in a section level represent an arbitrary cut-off between micrometastases and isolated tumor cells. The clinical significance of *isolated tumor cells* or *tumor cell groups* (≤ 0.2 mm or < 200 cells per cutting level, **Fig. 9.8**) seems to be minimal, if any.

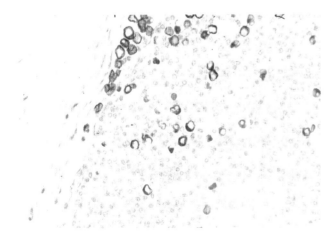

Fig. 9.7

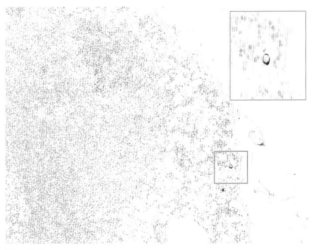

Fig. 9.8

The next most powerful prognostic factor is *the size of the tumor*, defined as *the largest dimension of the largest invasive focus*. Survival of the patients having, mammographically detected < 15 mm invasive carcinoma is not significantly different from that of women not having breast carcinoma (see also Chapters 2, 7, and 8).

The TNM tumor classification system used by the oncologists accepts measuring the tumor size primarily on macroscopic examination.

The macroscopic size of the largest invasive focus correlates very closely with both the mammographic size and the tumor size as measured on breast ultrasound (**Fig. 9.10**). These methods evaluate the central body of the tumor,

which is a parameter representative of tumor cell mass and which correlates with patient survival (**Fig. 9.11**). Magnetic resonance imaging has a tendency to slightly overestimate the size of the tumor measuring together the invasive component and (part of) the in situ component of the tumor. A histological large section taken in the plane of the largest tumor dimension provides medical documentation (**Fig. 9.9**) of the tumor size allowing retrospective and reproducible measurement. It also allows detection of small invasive foci and other lesions that are not visible on macroscopic or radiological examinations. Comparison of mammographic, ultrasonographic, macroscopic, and histological tumor size is essential when determining the real size of the tumor.

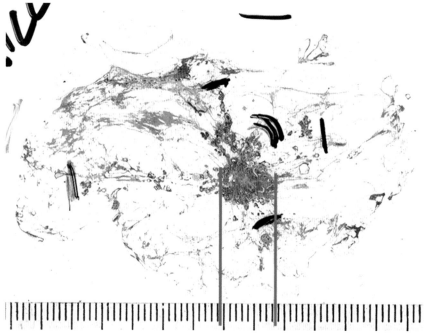

Fig. 9.9

Fig. 9.10

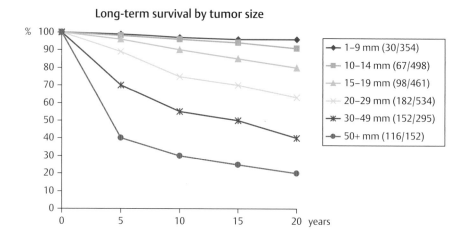

Long-term survival by tumor size

- 1–9 mm (30/354)
- 10–14 mm (67/498)
- 15–19 mm (98/461)
- 20–29 mm (182/534)
- 30–49 mm (152/295)
- 50+ mm (116/152)

Fig. 9.11

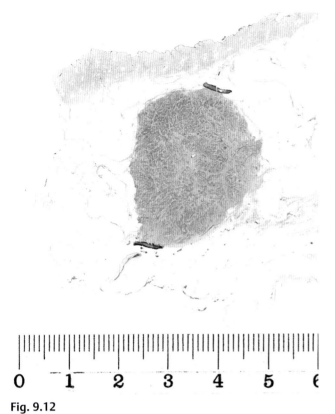

Fig. 9.12

Fig. 9.13

In cases of round or oval tumors (**Fig. 9.12**) the comparison is relatively easy and usually without discrepancies. In cases of stellate tumors, however, the tumor body should be measured histologically without the spiculations; otherwise the histological size becomes disproportionately larger as compared with the mammographic or ultrasonographic measurements or macroscopic size. The spiculations contain a relatively low number of tumor cells, and they do not represent a prognostically important aspect of the tumor.

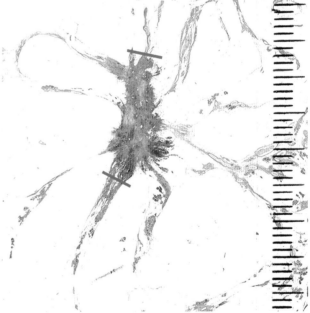

Fig. 9.14

The tumors in **Figs. 9.12, 9.13,** and **9.14** are not the same size, although if the spiculations (extensions) are measured and included, both tumors would measure 30 mm. The correct way to histologically assess tumor size is demonstrated in **Fig. 9.14**, compared with the erroneous assessment in **Fig. 9.13**.

In cases with multiple invasive tumor foci, the size of each tumor focus is measured separately, but for TNM classification only the largest focus size is recorded. Diffuse invasive breast carcinomas are adequately characterized by their extent.

Fig. 9.15 demonstrates the suggested way of measuring the size of the tumors of different shapes and in case of multifocality and diffuse invasion.

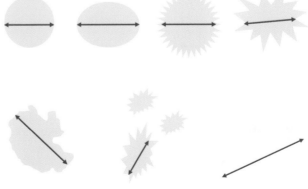

Fig. 9.15

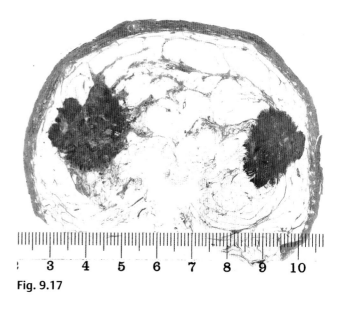

Fig. 9.16

Fig. 9.17

Multifocality of the invasive component, as defined in Chapter 2, carries important prognostic information. This category includes all tumors with multiple simultaneous invasive tumor foci within the same breast irrespective of whether they are localized within the same (**Fig. 9.16**) or in different quadrants (so-called multicentric cancers, **Fig. 9.17**). As seen in **Fig. 9.18**, the disease-specific survival of these patients is significantly worse compared with those having unifocal tumors. Patients with diffuse invasive carcinomas are few in number (**Fig. 9.19**) but have the worst outcome (see Chapter 10, Cases 2, 4, and 9).

Patients with invasive carcinomas showing a complex growth pattern with both focal and diffuse invasion (**Fig. 9.20**) share the unfavorable prognosis of those having purely diffuse invasive cancers.

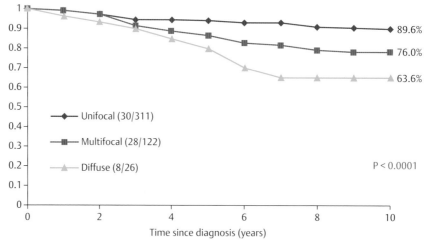

Fig. 9.18 Cumulative disease-specific survival in 459 consecutive invasive breast carcinoma cases by distribution of the invasive component. Dalarna County, Sweden, 1996–1998. (Reproduced from reference 7 with permission of the publisher.)

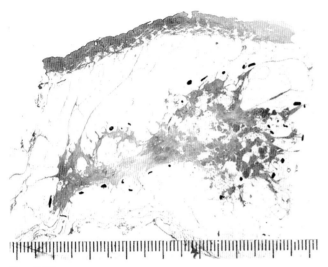

Fig. 9.19

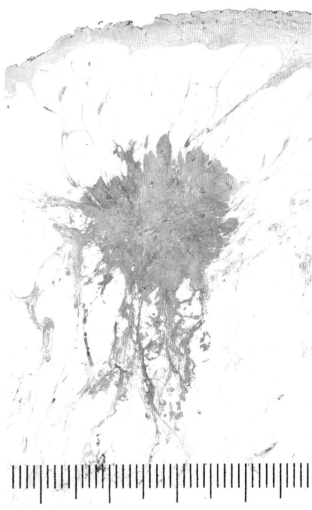

Lymph node metastases in multifocal invasive cancers are twice as frequent as in unifocal cancers; the corresponding ratio for diffuse invasive breast cancers is threefold. These differences are related to large-volume macrometastatic disease in multifocal and diffuse cases and are independent of the size, grade, or molecular phenotype of the tumors (see Chapter 10, Cases 2, 4, and 9).

The aggregate growth pattern (combined distribution of the in situ and invasive tumor components, as defined in Chapter 2) also carries prognostic information. As shown in **Fig. 9.21**, patients with cancers having multifocal and diffuse aggregate growth patterns had a poorer survival than those having unifocal cancers.

Fig. 9.20

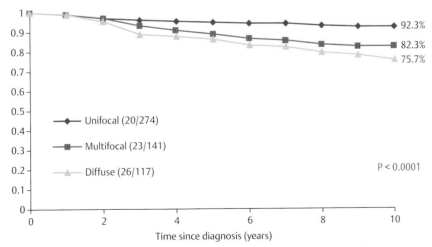

Fig. 9.21 Cumulative disease-specific survival in 532 consecutive invasive breast carcinoma cases by combined (in situ + invasive) lesion distribution. Dalarna County, Sweden, 1996–1998. (Reproduced from reference 7 with permission of the publisher.)

The *extent of the disease* (the area or tissue volume including all the malignant structures within the breast) is approximated by measuring in two or three dimensions as distances between the most distant tumor cells irrespective of whether the cells are in an in situ portion of the tumor, within an invasive tumor, or in its spiculations or in the lumen of a close lymph vessel. As mentioned in Chapter 2, *breast carcinomas of limited extent* (extent < 40 mm in largest dimension, **Fig. 9.16**) are appropriate candidates for breast-conserving surgery.

On the other hand, *extensive breast carcinomas* (**Fig. 9.23**) with a greater distance between invasive or in situ tumor foci and with extent 40 mm or more in largest dimension represent a risk for insufficient surgical intervention and local tumor recurrence.

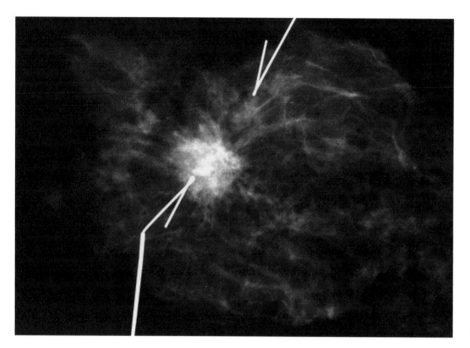

Fig. 9.22

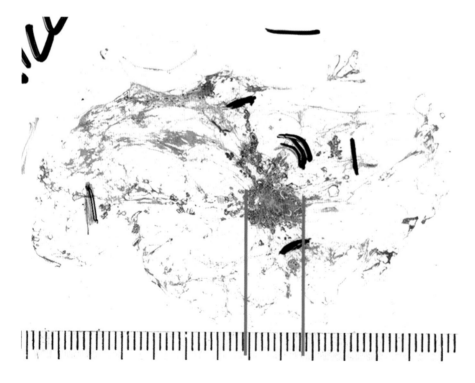

Fig. 9.23

As mentioned previously, the radiologically and the histologically determined disease extents are concordant in the vast majority of cases, but they may substantially deviate from each other in the presence of radiologically occult noncalcified ductal carcinoma in situ (DCIS) (**Figs. 9.22** and **9.23**, see also Chapter 10, Case 5), lobular carcinoma in situ (LCIS), or small invasive tumor foci.

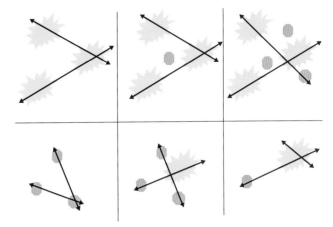

Fig. 9.24

Figs. **9.24** and **9.25** demonstrate the suggested method of measuring the extent of disease in cancers with multifocal and diffuse aggregate growth patterns. The blue color indicates the structure of the invasive component, the orange color indicates the structure of the in situ component of the tumors.

As illustrated in **Fig. 9.26**, disease extent is also a significant prognostic parameter in terms of disease-specific cumulative survival.

Fig. 9.25

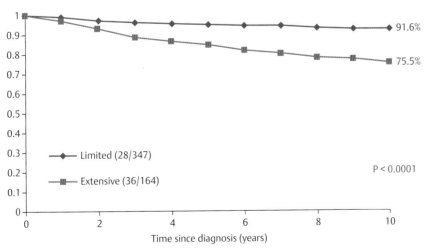

Fig. 9.26 Cumulative disease-specific survival in 511 consecutive breast carcinoma cases by disease extent. Limited: tumors occupying an area less than 40 mm in the largest dimension. Extensive: tumors occupying an area 40 mm or more in the largest dimension. (Reproduced from reference 7 with permission of the publisher.)

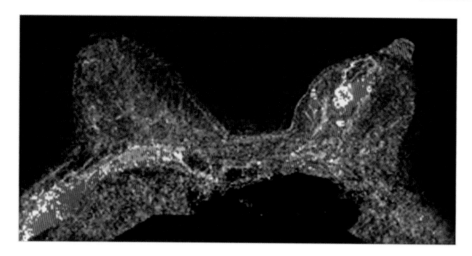

Fig. 9.27

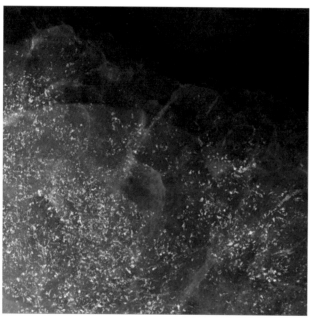

Fig. 9.28

The *grade and especially the extent of the associated ductal carcinoma in situ* are also well-recognized prognostic factors for cases of invasive cancer. **Fig. 9.27** is a magnetic resonance imaging study of one such case with foci of invasive tumor component (color mapped in red and yellow) and an extensive diffuse DCIS occupying a whole lobe (color mapped in blue). Invasive tumors associated with extensive DCIS grade III have a significantly less favorable prognosis than the tumors without extensive DCIS or with extensive DCIS grade I. As mentioned in Chapter 4, DCIS grade III is often associated with "casting type" microcalcifications on the mammogram (**Fig. 9.28**), which is a powerful mammographic prognostic parameter (**Fig. 9.29**) (see Chapter 10, Cases 3 and 10).

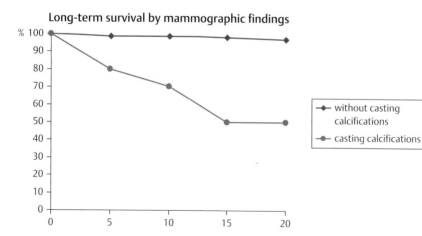

Long-term survival by mammographic findings

— without casting calcifications

— casting calcifications

Fig. 9.29 (Reproduced from reference 4 with permission of the publisher.)

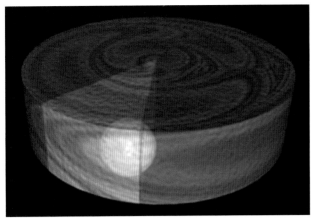

Fig. 9.30

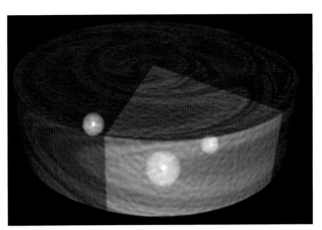

Fig. 9.31

The aim of the surgical intervention is often defined as excising the tumor with free margins. Failure to completely excise the tumor increases the risk of local recurrences and also indicates the need for completing surgery. The recommended width of the tumor-free margin varies considerably in different guidelines, the minimum being "no tumor at the ink," which may mean less than a millimeter margin. The advantages of large-section histology in assessing the margins were discussed in Chapter 8. Although the circumferential surgical margin is regularly documented in one plane in a large section (Fig. 9.32), small blocks are often needed to document the deep and superficial margins (Fig. 9.33).

Although removing a unifocal tumor with free margins is relatively easy, seemingly free surgical margins may be created in between the foci of a multifocal tumor. Failure of the surgical intervention in these two settings is illustrated in Figs. 9.30 and 9.31.

Shifting the aim of the surgical intervention from excising the tumor with free margins to excising the entire tissue at risk of developing cancer (the sick lobe) resulted in the concept of sector resection (segmentectomy). Excising a lobe is very difficult because of the complex interrelation of the lobes and the lack of anatomical borders between them. Despite this fact, this approach represents the standard method of breast-conserving surgery in many institutions ensuring low local recurrence rates and good cosmetic outcomes, especially if guided by detailed preoperative radiological mapping of the disease.

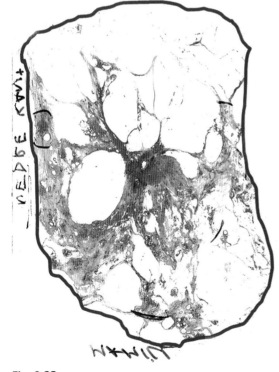

Fig. 9.32

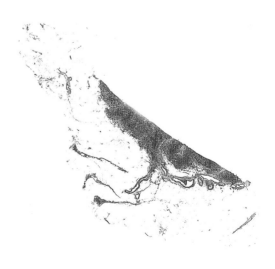

Fig. 9.33

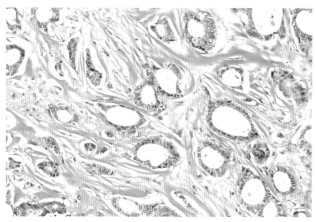

Fig. 9.34

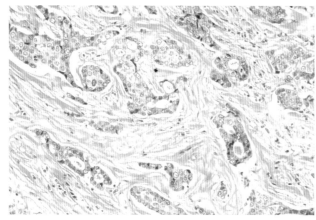

Fig. 9.35

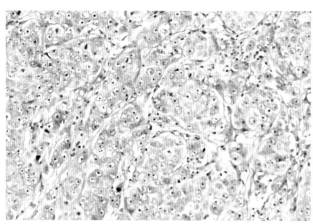

Fig. 9.36

The *malignancy grade* of the invasive carcinoma is a powerful prognostic factor in tumors larger than 10 (15) mm. It can be reproducibly evaluated by using the grading system of Bloom and Richardson, as modified by Elston. This system provides a score (ranging from 3 to 9 points), which sums up the assessment of the tubular structures, the nuclear grade, and the mitotic activity in a representative part of the tumor as follows:

Score 3–5:   grade I, well differentiated

Score 6–7:   grade II, intermediately differentiated

Score 8–9:   grade III, poorly differentiated

Tubular structures (tubule formation) are lumina surrounded by one or more layers of epithelial cells. The assessment is as follows:

– Tubules in more than 75% of the tumor	1 (**Fig. 9.34**)
– Tubules in 10% to 75% of the tumor	2 (**Fig. 9.35**)
– Tubules in less than 10% of the tumor	3 (**Fig. 9.36**)

The assessment of the *nuclear grade* is similar to the nuclear grading of DCIS. The assessment is as follows:

– Small, uniform nuclei	1 (**Fig. 9.38**)
– Larger nuclei with visible nucleoli, moderate variability in size and shape	2 (**Fig. 9.40**)
– Large, vesicular nuclei with prominent nucleoli and marked variation in size and shape	3 (**Fig. 9.42**)

Mitotic figures are counted per 10 high-power fields at the tumor periphery. Only typical mitotic figures should be counted. The score depends on the field diameter of the microscope used, and the cut-off points have to be adjusted according to the optical parameters.

In this grading system, the tubular structures are relatively easy to assess. Careful counting of mitotic figures is a necessary part of the assessment. However, the nuclear grade is the least reproducible parameter of the system. The grading can be assisted with computer-guided image analysis, which is demonstrated in **Figs. 9.37, 9.39,** and **9.41**. The normal epithelial cell nuclei (dark blue column left) are compared with nuclei assessed as nuclear grade I (**Fig. 9.38**), grade II (**Fig. 9.40**), or grade III (**Fig. 9.42**). The higher nuclear grade contains not only large but also more polymorphous nuclei.

A simple way to reach higher intraobserver and interobserver agreement is to compare the diameter of the tumor cell nuclei with a histological detail of constant diameter (e.g., a red blood cell or a lymphocyte). In cases of nuclear grade I, the tumor nuclei should not have a diameter larger than about two erythrocytes. In grade III, however, tumor cell nuclei with diameters larger than three erythrocytes occur frequently.

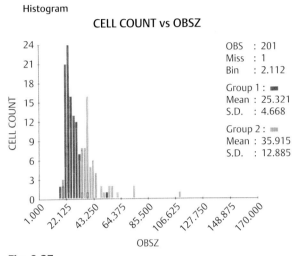

Fig. 9.37

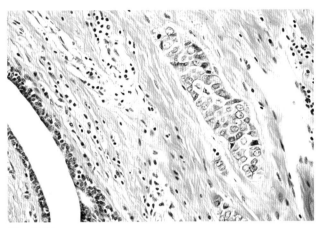

Fig. 9.38

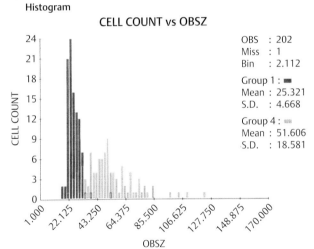

Fig. 9.39

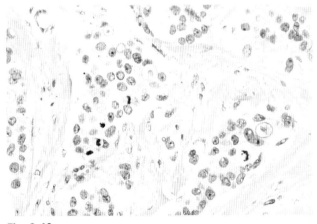

Fig. 9.40

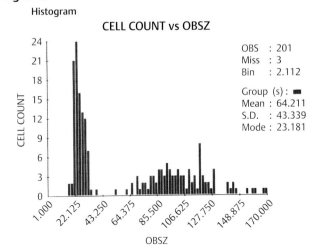

Fig. 9.41

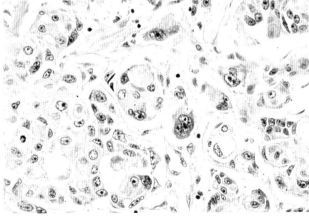

Fig. 9.42

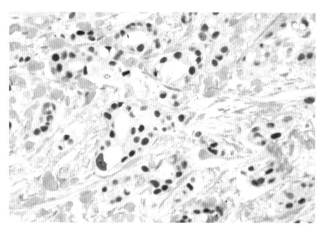

Fig. 9.43

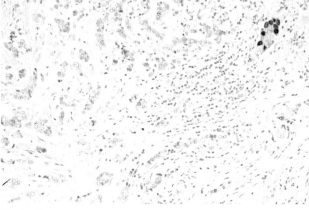

Fig. 9.44

Estrogen and progesterone receptor status is a prognostic factor as well as a therapeutic one. Expression of the receptors by tumor cell nuclei indicates that the tumor has a high sensitivity to antihormonal therapy.

Hormone receptors are preferably demonstrated and assessed by immunohistochemistry on a histological section containing tumor tissue and surrounding normal epithelial structures. Automation and external quality control of immunostaining may enhance the reproducibility of the results. Although most of the tumors are obviously receptor-positive (**Fig. 9.43**), it is necessary to count the ratio of positively stained nuclei to all tumor cell nuclei in some cases. The proposed cut-off point for positivity is 10%. A negative staining result can be accepted only in the presence of positive controls, preferably the nuclei of the normal tissue in the same section (**Fig. 9.44**). Normal mammary glands always exhibit estrogen and progesterone receptor-positivity but never in 100% of the epithelial cells.

Proliferative activity of the tumor cells is a very sensitive prognostic parameter. Breast carcinomas with high proliferative activity (**Fig. 9.45**) are rapidly growing tumors often detected during the interval between two screening events and are associated with a poor prognosis

(see Chapter 10, Case 7). The proliferative activity of the tumor is most often assessed by immunohistochemistry using the Ki67 index counted as percentage of the tumor cells expressing this marker in a "hot spot" (highest staining region at low-power microscopic magnification). Despite its frequent intratumoral heterogeneity, the difficulties in choosing the hot spots for counting, the poor interobserver reproducibility, and the lack of an internationally accepted cut-off value, high Ki67 index has become one of the basic parameters for recommending chemotherapy. Several guidelines recommend a cut-off of 20% to delineate cancers with high and intermediate/low proliferative activity (**Fig. 9.46**). A simple way of enhancing reproducibility of the assessment of Ki67 staining (after counting 200 or 300 tumor cells) is to check the result judging the density of the staining as follows:

more than half of the nuclei stained = very high proliferation

more than a third of nuclei stained = high proliferation

about every fourth or fifth nucleus stained = borderline case (count carefully)

less than a fifth of the cells stained = low or intermediate proliferation.

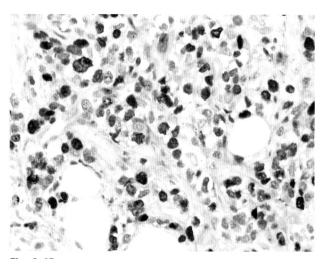

Fig. 9.45

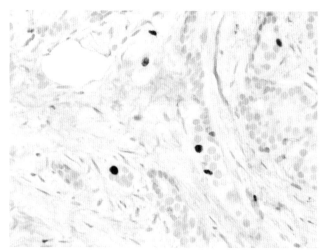

Fig. 9.46

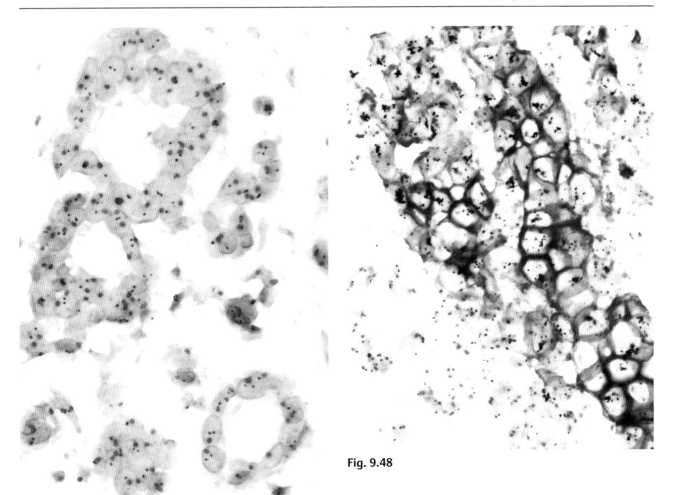

Fig. 9.48

Fig. 9.47

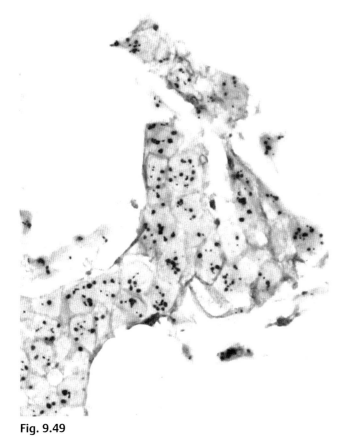

Expression of c-erbB-2 oncogene (HER2) in the tumor is associated with poorer survival of the patients. HER2 expressing cells are the target of the specific therapy with an antibody against this protein called trastuzumab. Proper assessment of HER2 expression is therefore essential. The method of dual silver in situ hybridization demonstrates the centromere of chromosome 17 (red dots) and the copies of HER2 gene (black dots) in the nuclei. Expression of HER2 protein in the cell membrane can also be visualized within the same slide (brown stain). A HER2-negative case (**Fig. 9.47**) is characterized with an equal number (usually two and two) of red and black dots in the nuclei and absent or weak staining of the membrane ("0 or 1+"). The tumor cells in a HER2-positive case (**Fig. 9.48**) exhibit strong and complete circumferential membranous staining in > 10% of the tumor cells ("3+") and a HER2 gene/centromere-17 copy number index > 2. In cases with high amplification, the copies of the HER2 gene often appear in clusters. Using this technique, indeterminate cases (**Fig. 9.49**) will be few and often related to polysomy of chromosome 17.

Fig. 9.49

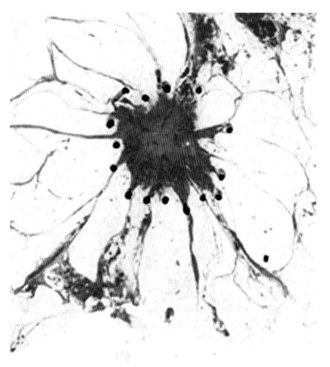

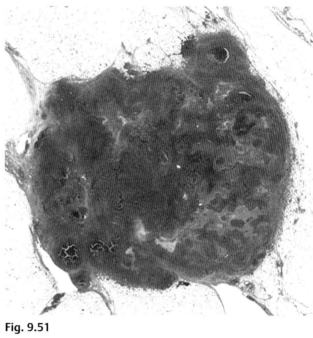

Fig. 9.51

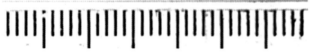

Fig. 9.50

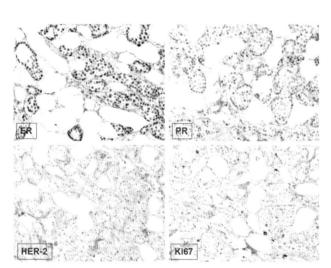

Fig. 9.52

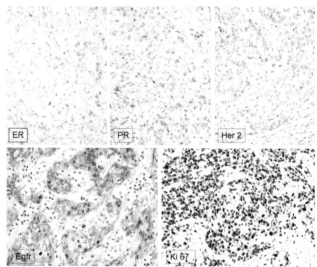

Fig. 9.53

Table 9.1 Invasive breast carcinomas by size, shape, and some molecular characteristics, Dalarna County, Sweden, 2008–2012

	Luminal A	Basal-like	HER2-positive	Triple negative	Grade 3
Stellate <15 mm	92% (171/185)	3% (5/185)	4% (8/185)	2% (4/185)	2% (4/185)
Stellate ≥15 mm	85% (215/252)	6% (15/252)	9% (24/252)	1% (2/252)	15% (37/252)
Circular <15 mm	79% (100/127)	8% (10/127)	10% (13/127)	9% (11/127)	17% (22/127)
Circular ≥15 mm	58% (113/196)	29% (56/196)	16% (32/196)	21% (41/196)	43% (84/196)

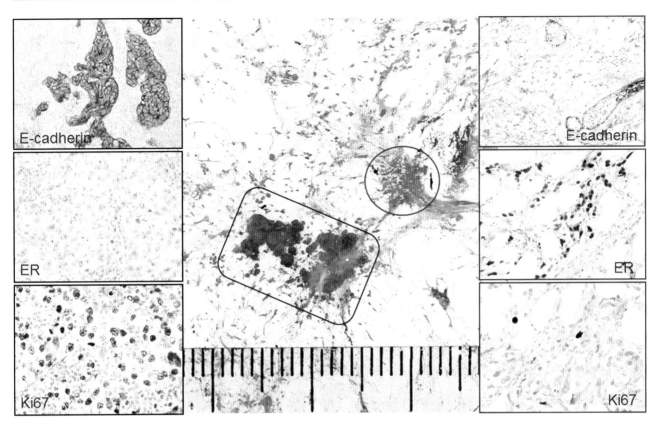

Fig. 9.54

The genetic construction of breast carcinomas can be traced with sufficient accuracy using immunohistochemistry. The tumors are classified into Luminal A, Luminal B, HER2 type, and basal-like molecular phenotype categories. Luminal A tumors express estrogen receptors but do not express basal markers and HER-2 (**Figs. 9.50** and **9.52**). The vast majority of patients with such tumors have a good prognosis, but exceptions exist (e.g. diffuse invasive lobular carcinomas). The Luminal B category is defined in the literature as estrogen receptor -positive tumors with either high proliferative activity, or high grade, or HER2 expression, or low levels of progesterone receptor expression. Similarly, there is a lack of consensus in defining the basal-like category: in some classifications, these tumors correspond to triple-negative cancers lacking expression of both estrogen and progesterone receptors and HER2. In other systems these tumors are delineated on the basis of expression of "basal" markers (such as cytokeratin 5, cytokeratin 14, or epithelial growth factor receptor [EGFR]) otherwise typical of the normal myoepithelium (see Chapter 10, Case 8). Additional molecular phenotypes such as "claudin low" or "molecular apocrine" have been recently described.

Table 9.1 demonstrates a clear interrelation between the radiological and oncological prognostic parameters. Although the small stellate tumors exhibit favorable molecular and histological characteristics in the vast majority of cases, the large circular/oval masses represent high-grade and/or basal-like carcinomas much more often.

Our simple practical approach divides breast carcinomas into estrogen receptor positive and estrogen receptor negative tumors. The estrogen receptor positive tumors are further divided into Luminal A (not expressing HER2) and Luminal B (expressing HER2) categories. The estrogen receptor–negative tumors are further divided into HER2 type (expressing HER2) and triple negative (not expressing HER2 and progesterone receptors). Any tumor expressing at least one of the "basal" markers is classified as basal-like breast cancer (**Figs. 9.51** and **9.53**). Tumors expressing estrogen receptors have excellent prognosis, tumors not expressing estrogen receptors have an intermediate prognosis, whereas basal-like tumors have the worst outcome.

The individual invasive foci of a multifocal breast carcinoma may deviate from each other in tumor type, histology grade, or molecular phenotype. Such intertumoral heterogeneity is seen in up to 30% of multifocal cancers and may influence the therapeutic decisions and the tumors' response to the therapy. Intratumoral heterogeneity is also seen relatively often, especially on the genetic level, and has a similar impact. **Fig. 9.54** illustrates a multifocal cancer with two foci very close to each other but showing divergent molecular phenotypes.

Long-term survival by histological types and grade

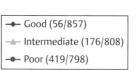

Good (56/857)
Intermediate (176/808)
Poor (419/798)

Fig. 9.55 (Reproduced from reference 4 with permission of the publisher.)

Conclusions

By assessing the main morphological–prognostic parameters described in this chapter, the many variations of breast carcinoma can be stratified into the following three categories in terms of breast cancer specific survival and overall survival, as shown in **Fig. 9.55**:

– Breast cancer cases with a good prognosis—most in situ carcinomas, early invasive carcinomas (smaller than 15 mm), tubular carcinomas, and mucinous carcinomas

– Breast cancer cases with a poor prognosis—tumors with metastases, diffuse invasive carcinomas, tumors having an in situ component with neoductgenesis, and tumors larger than 20 mm

– Breast cancer cases with an intermediate prognosis

Local recurrence is related to the extent and multifocality of the tumor as well as to the radicality of the previous surgical intervention.

Bibliography

1. Lakhani SR, Ellis IO, Schnitt SJ et al. eds. WHO Classification of Tumors of the Breast. Lyon, France: International Agency for Research on Cancer; 2012
2. Perry N, Puthaar E; *European Commission. Directorate-General for Health and Consumer Protection,* et al. European Guidelines for Quality Assurance in Breast Cancer Screening and Diagnosis. 4th ed. Luxembourg, Belgium; Office for Official Publications of the European Communities; 2006:222–248
3. Elston CW, Ellis JO. Pathological prognostic factors in breast cancer, I: The value of histological grade in breast cancer: experience from a large study with long-term follow-up. Histopathology 1991;19(5):403–410
4. Tabár L, Vitak B, Chen HH, et al. The Swedish Two-County Trial twenty years later: updated mortality results and new insights from long-term follow-up. Radiol Clin North Am 2000;38(4):625–651
5. Faverly DRG, Hendriks JHCL, Holland R. Breast carcinomas of limited extent: frequency, radiologic-pathologic characteristics, and surgical margin requirements. Cancer 2001;91(4):647–659
6. Tabár L, Tony Chen HH, Amy Yen MF, et al. Mammographic tumor features can predict long-term outcomes reliably in women with 1-14-mm invasive breast carcinoma. Cancer 2004;101(8):1745–1759
7. Tot T, Gere M, Pekár G, et al. Breast cancer multifocality, disease extent, and survival. Hum Pathol 2011;42(11):1761–1769
8. Tot T, Pekár G. Multifocality in "basal-like" breast carcinomas and its influence on lymph node status. Ann Surg Oncol 2011;18(6):1671–1677
9. Tot T. Early and more advanced unifocal and multifocal breast carcinomas and their molecular phenotypes. Clin Breast Cancer 2011;11(4):258–263
10. Lindquist D, Hellberg D, Tot T. Disease extent >=4 cm is a prognostic marker of local recurrence in T1-2 breast cancer. Pathol Res Int 2011;2011:860845
11. Tot T. Axillary lymph node status in unifocal, multifocal, and diffuse breast carcinomas: differences are related to macrometastatic disease. Ann Surg Oncol 2012;19(11):3395–3401

Chapter 10

Case Reports

Case 1. The Importance of Intratumoral Heterogeneity

An 80-year-old woman presented with a large, palpable, rapidly growing lump that filled her right breast (**Fig. 10.1.1**).

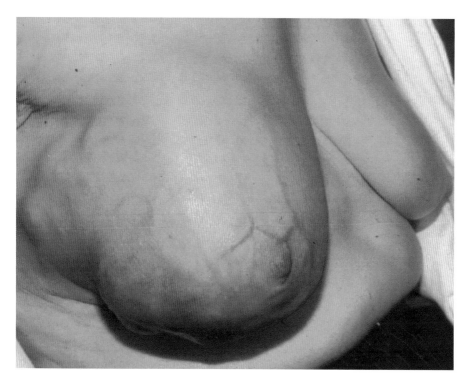

Fig. 10.1.1

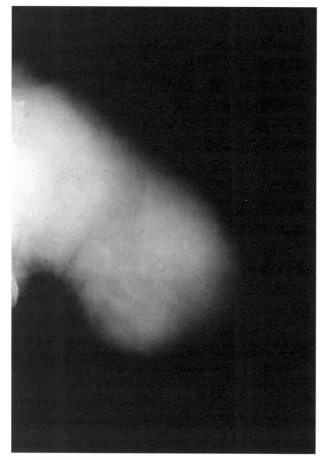

Mammography and ultrasonography demonstrated a large (7-cm) malignant tumor (**Figs. 10.1.2** and **10.1.3**).

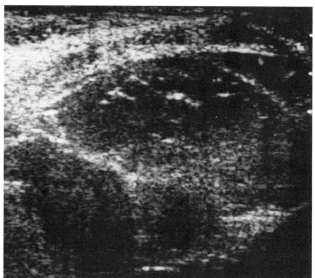

Fig. 10.1.2

Fig. 10.1.3

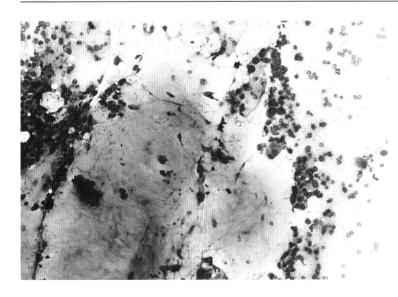

Fig. 10.1.4

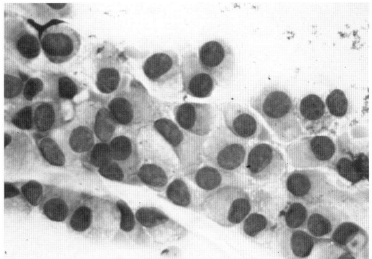

Fig. 10.1.5

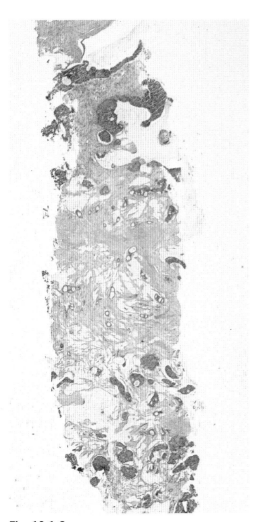

Fine-needle aspiration biopsy yielded a cellular smear with a mucinous background and cellular atypia (**Figs. 10.1.4** and **10.1.5**). A definitive preoperative diagnosis of invasive mucinous carcinoma was made by core biopsy (**Figs. 10.1.6** and **10.1.7**).

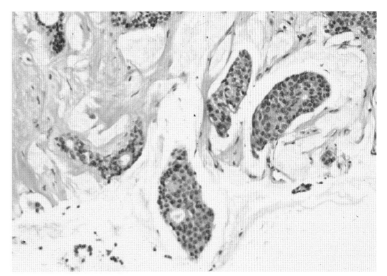

Fig. 10.1.6

Fig. 10.1.7

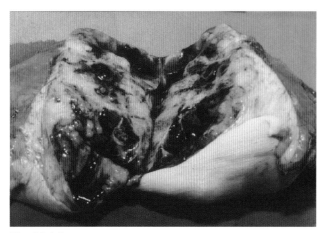

Fig. 10.1.8

Mastectomy was performed and a large tumor with a partly hemorrhagic cut surface was macroscopically evident (**Fig. 10.1.8**). On the histological large section, nearly the entire cut surface could be seen (**Fig. 10.1.9**). Almost 90% of the tumor exhibited the typical picture of mucinous carcinoma with groups of well-differentiated tumor cells floating in a large amount of mucin (**Fig. 10.1.10**). However, an area (~20 × 10 mm) of more solid tumor tissue was also evident (marked with arrow in **Fig. 10.1.9**).

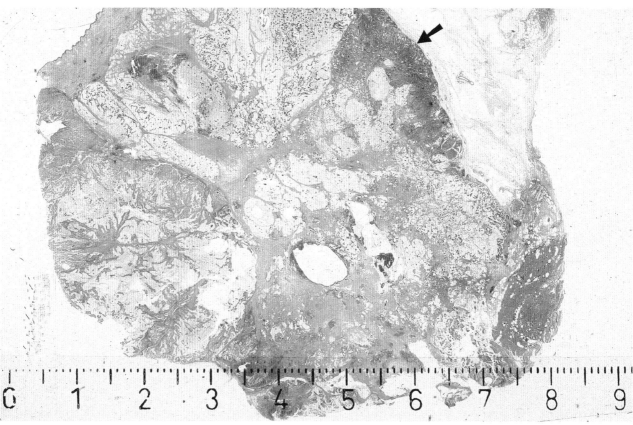

Fig. 10.1.9

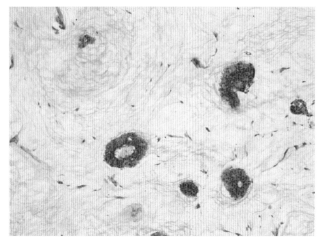

Fig. 10.1.10

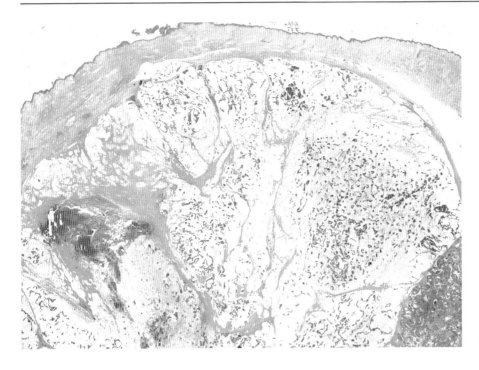

Fig. 10.1.11

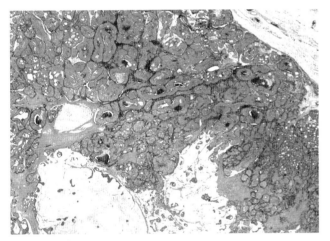

Fig. 10.1.12

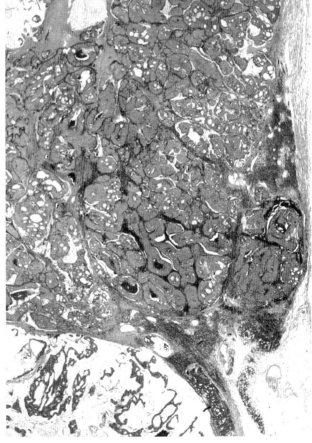

The solid part of the tumor was clearly different from the
mucinous component. The cells were poorly differentiated
and formed solid nests with central necrosis (Figs. 10.1.11 to
10.1.13). The pattern corresponds to a poorly differentiated,
grade III ductal carcinoma.

Fig. 10.1.13

The grade III component of the tumor infiltrated the pectoralis muscle (**Fig. 10.1.14**). Lymph vessel invasion was verified (**Fig. 10.1.15**), and the cancer had metastasized to one of the nine examined lymph nodes (**Fig. 10.1.16**).

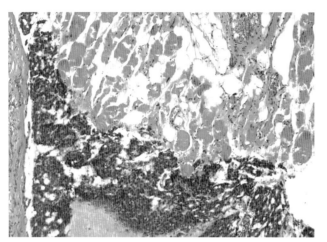

Fig. 10.1.14

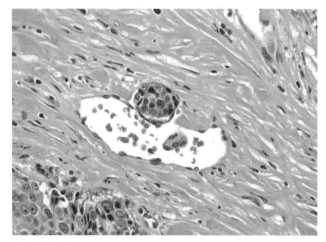

Fig. 10.1.15

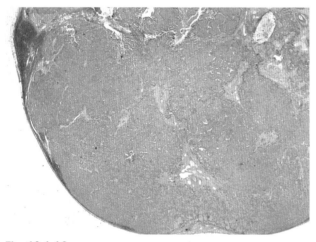

Fig. 10.1.16

Conclusions

Although the tumor fulfilled the criteria for mucinous carcinoma (grade I tumor with a mucinous pattern in 90% of the histological picture), the patient outcome will be determined by the minor grade III component (**Fig.10.1.17**).

A thorough postoperative workup should include a search for evidence of intratumoral heterogeneity.

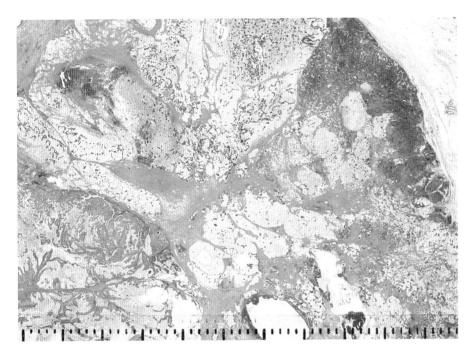

Fig. 10.1.17

Case 2. Unifocal Early Breast Cancer

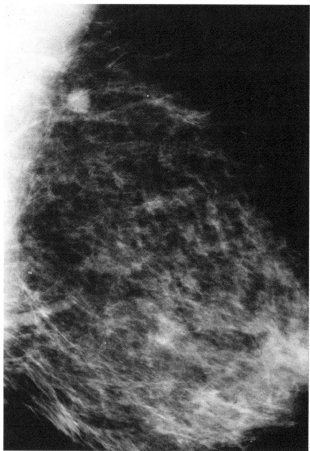

Fig. 10.2.1

A malignant breast lesion was detected by mammographic screening in a 56-year-old asymptomatic woman (**Fig. 10.2.1**). Ultrasound-guided fine-needle aspiration biopsy (FNAB) yielded a cellular smear without myoepithelial cells and with a large number of noncohesive epithelial cell groups (**Fig. 10.2.2**). The epithelial cells exhibited moderate atypia (**Fig. 10.2.3**). The preoperative cytological diagnosis was malignant breast tumor.

The large histological section (**Fig. 10.2.4**) demonstrated that the 7-mm tumor was unifocal invasive ductal carcinoma with an in situ component within the invasive area.

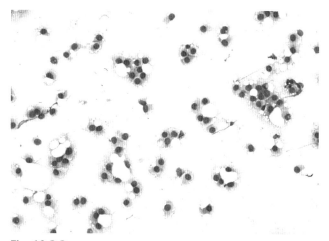

Fig. 10.2.2

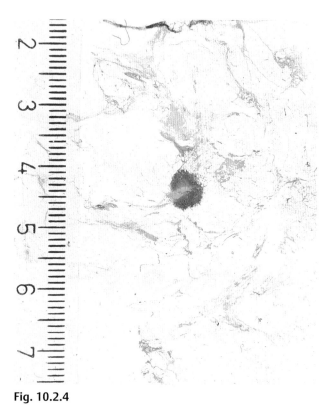

Fig. 10.2.4

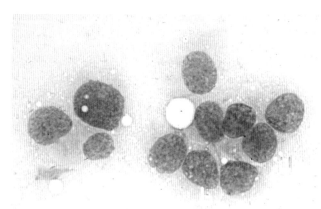

Fig. 10.2.3

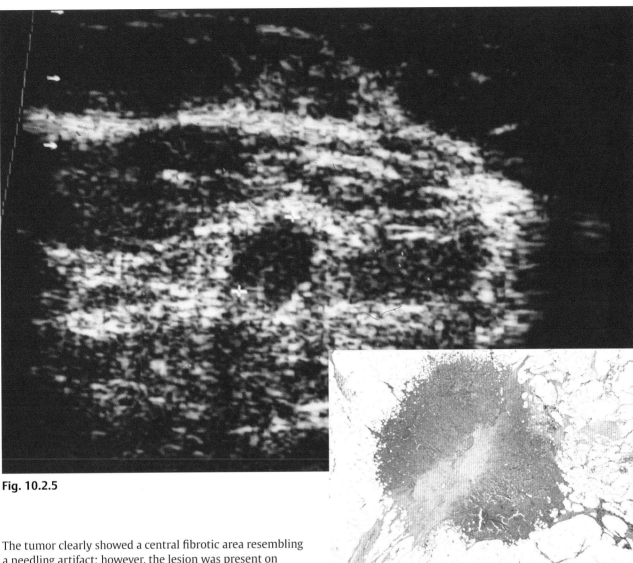

Fig. 10.2.5

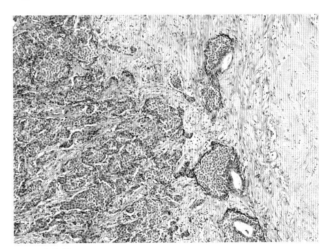

Fig. 10.2.6

The tumor clearly showed a central fibrotic area resembling a needling artifact; however, the lesion was present on ultrasound before the aspiration was performed (Figs. 10.2.5 and 10.2.6). The tumor was intermediately differentiated (Fig. 10.2.7), and the tumor cells were estrogen-receptor positive (Fig. 10.2.8).

The patient has been followed for 14 years and the tumor has not recurred.

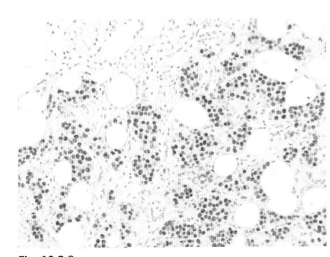

Fig. 10.2.8

Fig. 10.2.7

Conclusions

It is important to determine the size, distribution, and extent of the breast carcinoma because small, unifocal invasive carcinomas without an extensive in situ component have an excellent prognosis.

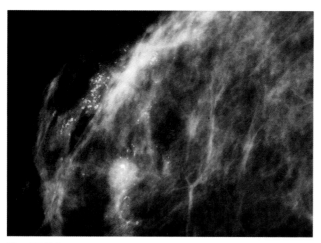

Fig. 10.3.1

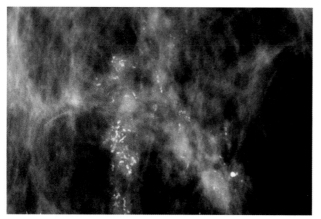

Fig. 10.3.2

Case 3. Extensive Breast Carcinoma

A 55-year-old woman presented with a mammographically detected nonpalpable tumor. In addition to the well-formed, small tumor mass, the mammogram showed a large area of microcalcifications of the casting type (**Figs. 10.3.1** and **10.3.2**). Core biopsy was performed and contained only structures of ductal carcinoma in situ (DCIS) (**Figs. 10.3.3** and **10.3.4**).

The correlation of mammographic and histological findings using the large-section technique revealed a large area of DCIS grade III. In this area, a 9-mm, grade III, invasive ductal carcinoma was also seen (**Figs. 10.3.5** and **10.3.6**).

The diagnosis of extensive ductal carcinoma grade III was established: the tumor size was 9 mm and the extent was 50 × 30 mm.

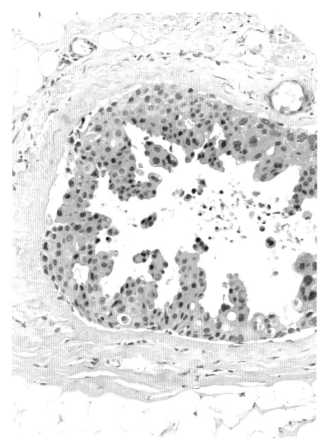

Fig. 10.3.4

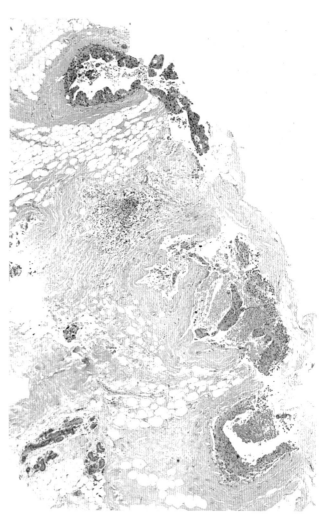

Fig. 10.3.3

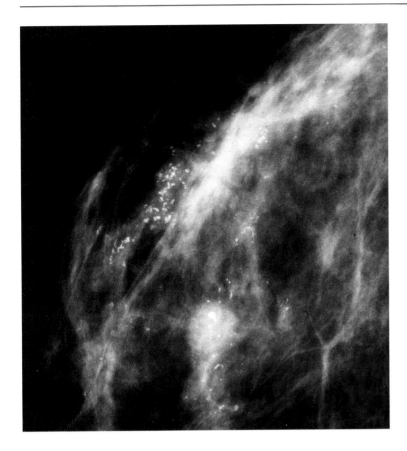

Fig. 10.3.5

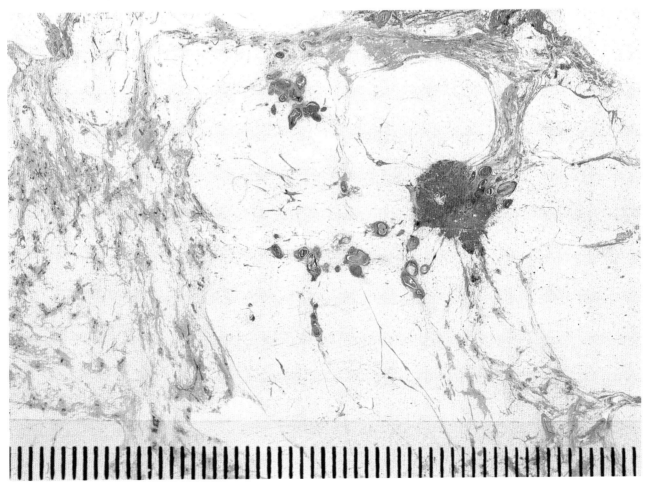

Fig. 10.3.6

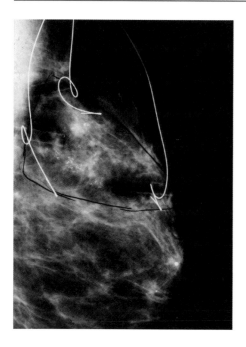

Fig. 10.3.7

Further details of the invasive and in situ component of the tumor are shown in **Figs. 10.3.7, 10.3.8, 10.3.9, 10.3.10, 10.3.11,** and **10.3.12**. The periductal inflammation and fibrosis, which are possible indirect signs of neoductgenesis, can be seen.

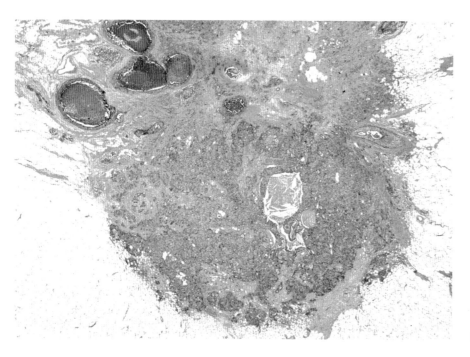

Fig. 10.3.8

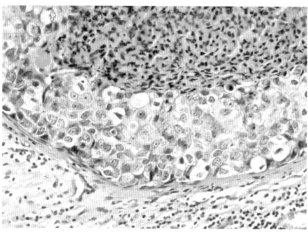

Fig. 10.3.9

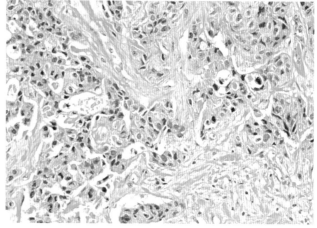

Fig. 10.3.10

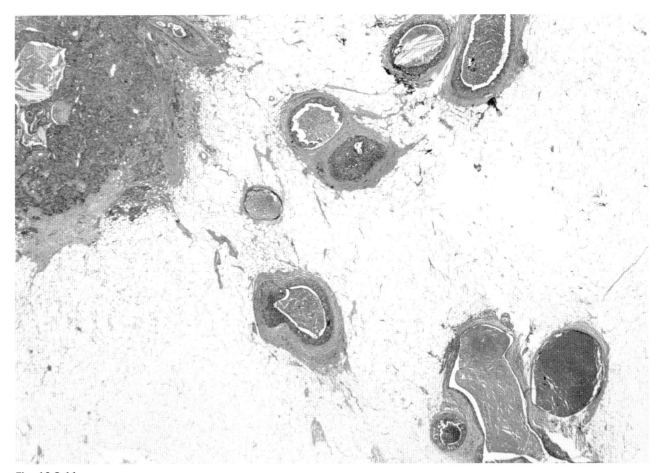

Fig. 10.3.11

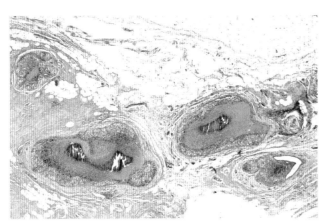

Fig. 10.3.12

As shown in **Fig. 10.3.13**, the patient had lymph node metastases in 3 of the 10 examined nodes. There have been no signs of recurrence during the follow-up period of 2 years.

Conclusions

Careful assessment of the extent of the disease is an important part of the postoperative workup because patients with extensive breast carcinomas, especially associated with grade III DCIS, have a worse prognosis than patients with breast carcinomas of the same size and grade but of limited extent (**Fig. 10.3.14**).

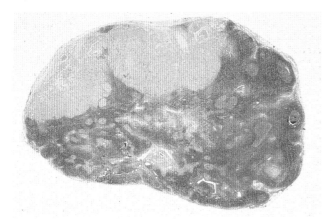

Fig. 10.3.13

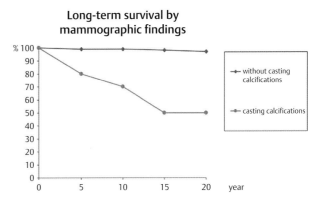

Fig. 10.3.14 (the same as **Fig. 9.17**)

Case 4. Extensive Invasive Lobular Carcinoma

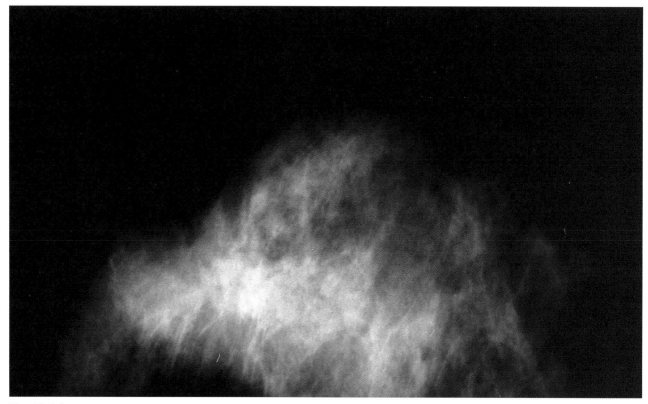

Fig. 10.4.1

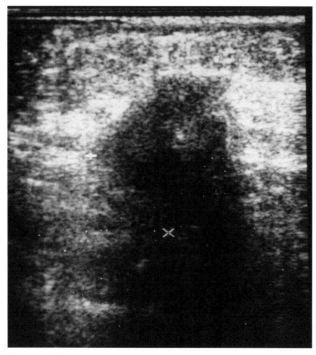

Fig. 10.4.2

This patient presented clinically with a large, diffuse, palpable lesion. Both the mammogram and the ultrasonographic examination demonstrated a large malignant tumor (**Figs. 10.4.1, 10.4.2,** and **10.4.8**). Fine-needle aspiration, however, yielded a smear with only a few groups of small, regular cells (**Fig. 10.4.3**).

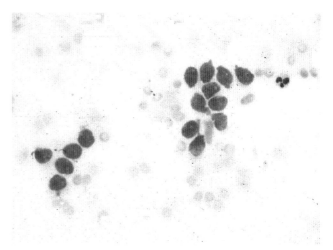

Fig. 10.4.3

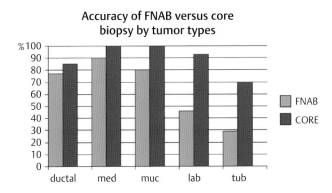

Fig. 10.4.4 (the same as Fig. 7.27)

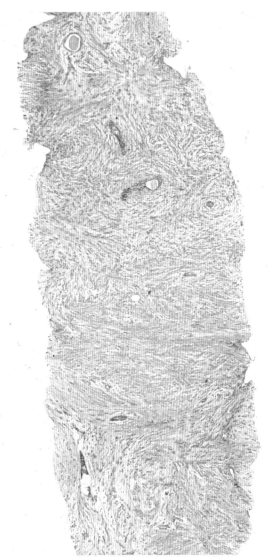

Core biopsy allowed the definitive preoperative diagnosis of invasive lobular carcinoma to be established (Figs. 10.4.5, 10.4.6, and 10.4.7). As discussed in Chapter 7, one of the advantages of core biopsy compared with FNAB is a higher accuracy in making the preoperative diagnosis of invasive lobular carcinoma (Fig. 10.4.4).

Fig. 10.4.5

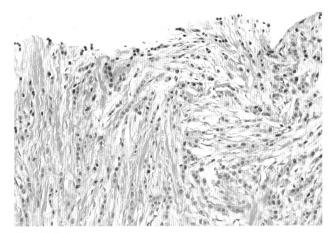

Fig. 10.4.6

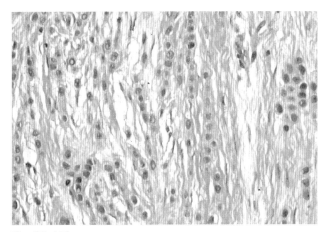

Fig. 10.4.7

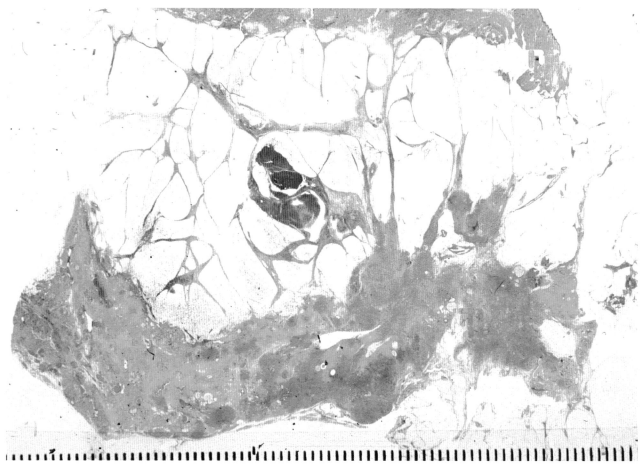

Fig. 10.4.8

Large-section histology (**Fig. 10.4.9**) showed an area of at least 50 × 30 mm of invasive lobular carcinoma, mainly of the classic type, with some intratumoral heterogeneity (**Figs. 10.4.10, 10.4.11,** and **10.4.12**). Four of the examined axillary lymph nodes contained metastases (**Fig. 10.4.13**). The patient died of metastatic breast carcinoma 3 years later.

Fig. 10.4.9

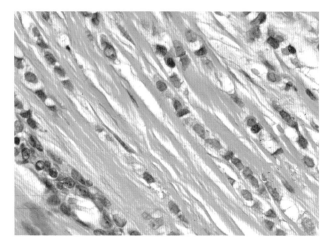

Fig. 10.4.10

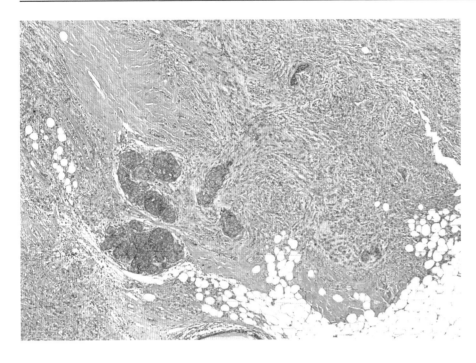

Fig. 10.4.11

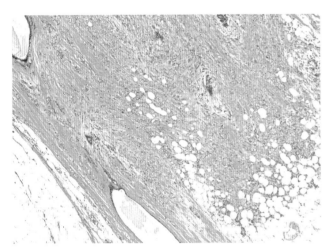

Fig. 10.4.12

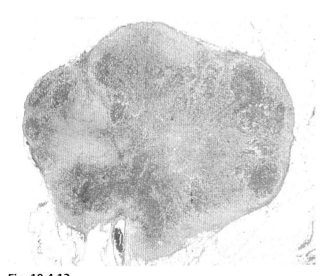

Fig. 10.4.13

Conclusions

Invasive lobular carcinoma may exhibit a diffuse growth pattern. These tumors are extensive, aggressive, and have a poor prognosis.

Case 5. Breast Carcinoma of Limited Extent

A 60-year-old asymptomatic woman presented with a unifocal stellate lesion detected by mammographic screening (**Fig. 10.5.1**), which was well visualized by ultrasonography (**Fig. 10.5.2**). The lesion was seen on the mammogram as a white star with a well-formed tumor body.

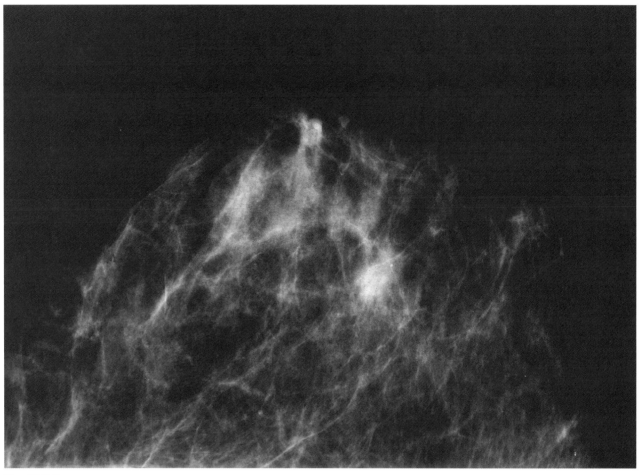

Fig. 10.5.1

Ultrasound-guided fine-needle aspiration was performed and yielded a moderately cellular smear with some cell groups with atypia (**Fig. 10.5.4**). The cytological picture was categorized as IV, suspicious for malignancy.

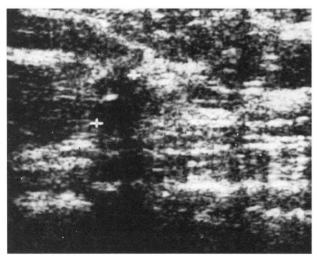

Fig. 10.5.2

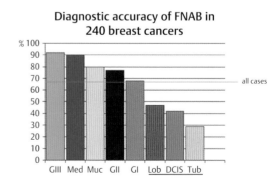

Fig. 10.5.3 (the same as **Fig. 7.21**)

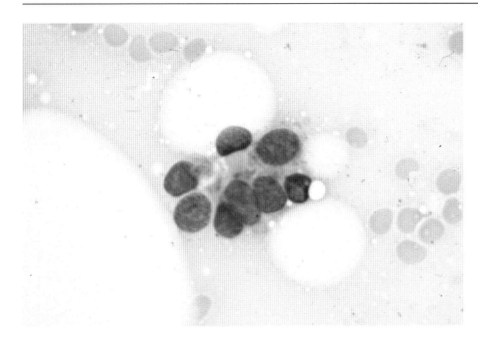

Fig. 10.5.4

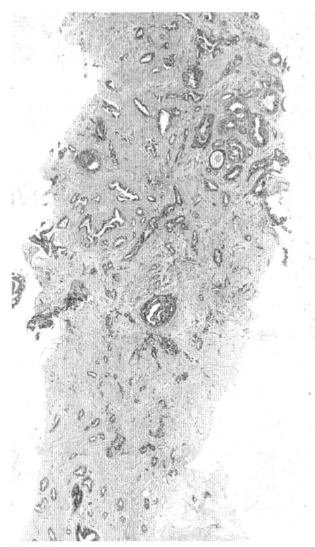

As mentioned in Chapter 7, FNAB is not an effective way of diagnosing tubular carcinoma (**Fig. 10.5.3**).

Preoperative core biopsy was indicated to confirm the malignant nature of the lesion. The core was representative and included tubular structures in an area of in situ carcinoma and normal structures (**Fig. 10.5.5**). To confirm the invasive character of the tubular structures, immunohistochemical staining on smooth muscle actin was performed (**Fig. 10.5.6**).

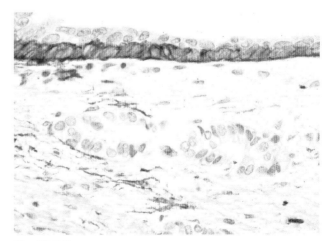

Fig. 10.5.5

Fig. 10.5.6

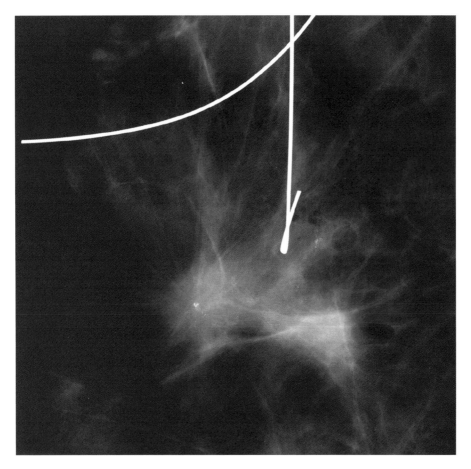

Fig. 10.5.7

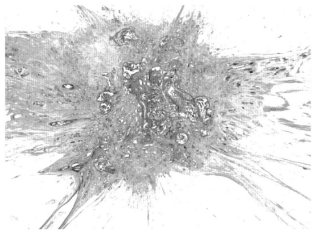

Fig. 10.5.8

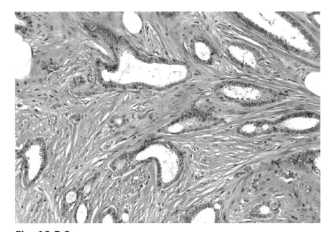

By correlating the mammographic findings with the findings on large-section histology, the solitary 8-mm stellate lesion could be easily recognized corresponding to invasive tubular carcinoma (Figs. 10.5.7, 10.5.8, 10.5.9, and 10.5.10) and containing structures of DCIS grade I within the tumor.

Fig. 10.5.9

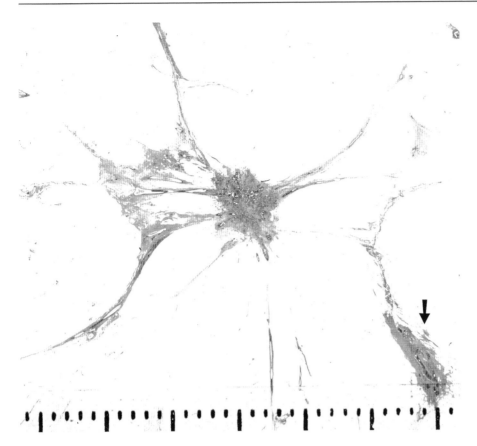

Fig. 10.5.10

Histology examination revealed a 3-mm focus fulfilling the criteria of DCIS grade I (**Fig. 10.5.10** and the corresponding magnification in **Fig. 10.5.11**) at a distance of 30 mm from the dominant tumor mass and very near the circumferential resection margin.

A completing surgical excision was done, but no tumor structures were detected in the excised tissue. There have been no signs of recurrence during the 13-year follow-up period.

Conclusions

This unifocal invasive tumor with a multifocal in situ component was of limited extent. Such tumors may be completely removed with sector resection.

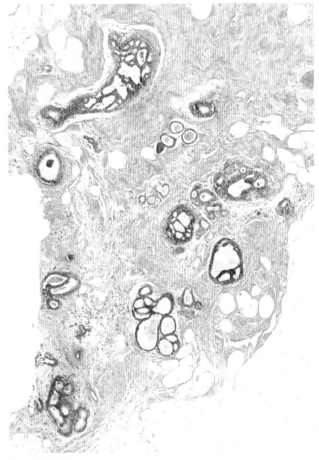

Fig. 10.5.11

Case 6. Tumor-forming DCIS

This 67-year-old woman noted a breast mass in her left breast. The radiological examination revealed a stellate tumor mass without signs of multifocality (**Fig. 10.6.1**). She also had palpable lymph nodes in her axilla.

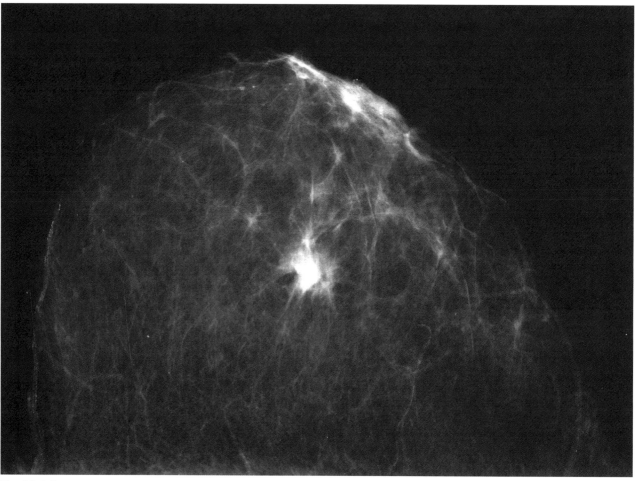

Fig. 10.6.1

FNAB yielded a cellular smear with moderate atypia and with a minimal number of myoepithelial cells, categorized as V, malignant (**Figs. 10.6.2** and **10.6.3**).

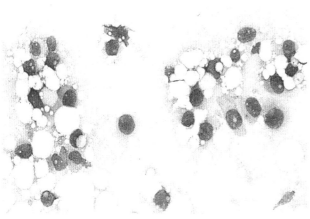

Fig. 10.6.2

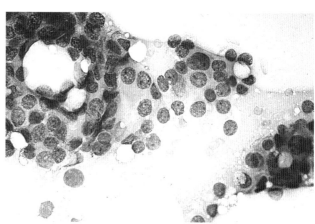

Fig. 10.6.3

Segmentectomy and axillary lymph node evacuation were performed. The large histological section (**Fig. 10.6.4**) demonstrated the solitary 10-mm lesion. At higher magnification (**Fig. 10.6.5**), epithelial displacement as a consequence of a needling procedure was well seen.

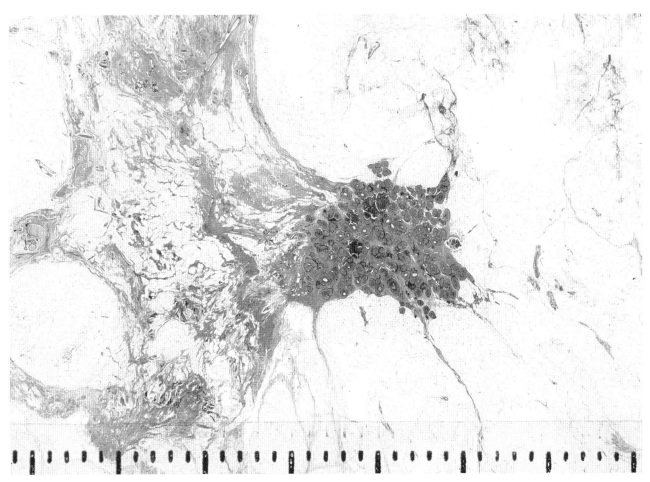

Fig. 10.6.4

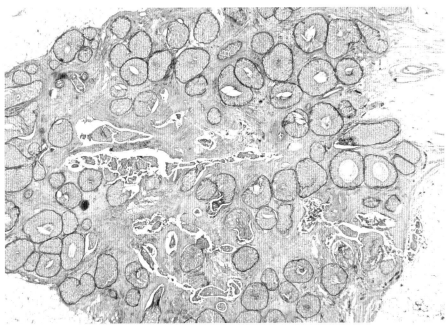

Fig. 10.6.5

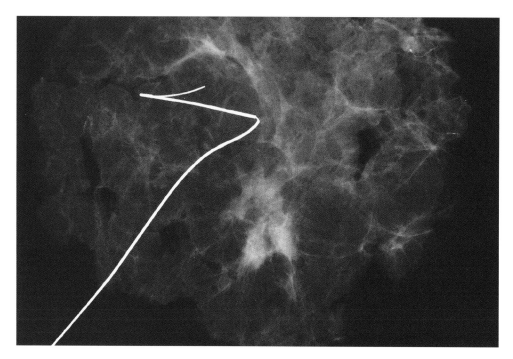

Fig. 10.6.6

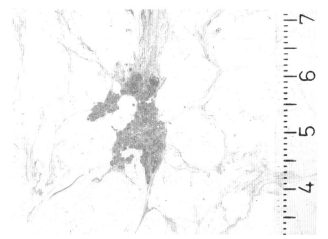

Fig. 10.6.7

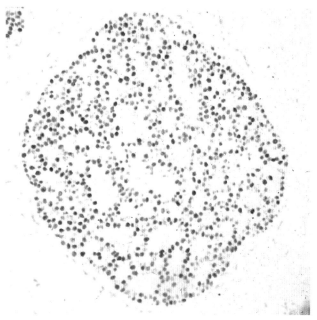

Fig. 10.6.8

In another slice of the tumor, the large section revealed that the tumor varied in size and shape (**Figs. 10.6.6** and **10.6.7**, as compared with **Fig. 10.6.4**). Pseudoinvasion, a consequence of the needling procedure, was also evident. However, the tumor structures had the form of dilated acini, and no invasion into the stroma could be demonstrated (**Fig. 10.6.8**). The basement membrane was also seen around the structures (**Figs. 10.6.9** and **10.6.10**). The lesion was diagnosed as ductal carcinoma in situ, grade I, tumor forming.

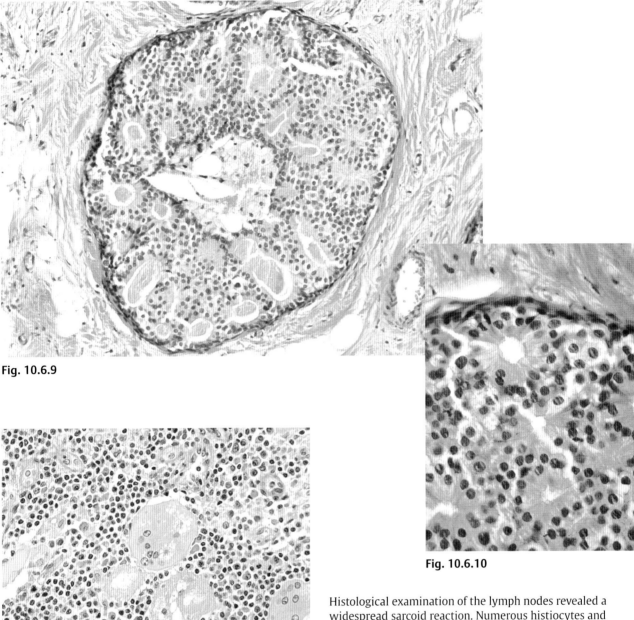

Fig. 10.6.9

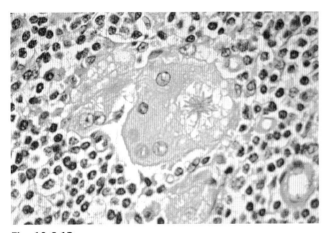

Fig. 10.6.10

Fig. 10.6.11

Histological examination of the lymph nodes revealed a widespread sarcoid reaction. Numerous histiocytes and multinucleated giant cells could be seen, some of which contained asteroid bodies (Figs. 10.6.11 and 10.6.12).

Conclusions

The rare tumor-forming subtype of DCIS often causes differential diagnostic difficulties. A sarcoid reaction, sometimes seen in lymph nodes draining tumors, may lead to a false clinical impression of the presence of lymph node metastasis.

Fig. 10.6.12

Case 7. Total Remission of Interval Cancer after Neoadjuvant Chemotherapy

This 51-year-old woman felt a 4-cm lump in her left breast 6 months after she had a negative screening mammography examination. Enlarged palpable lymph nodes were present in her left axilla.

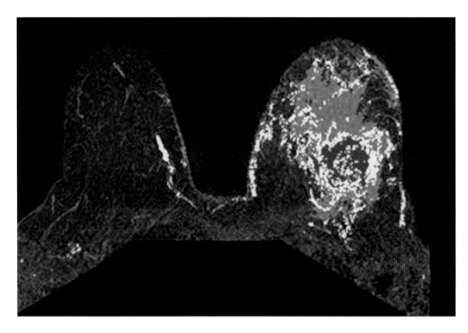

Fig. 10.7.1

In addition to mammography and breast ultrasound examination, magnetic resonance imaging was performed and revealed a round-shaped malignant tumor measuring 41 × 42 mm in the left breast. Persistent contrast enhancement on an area > 100 mm in the largest dimension was also seen surrounding the tumor and was interpreted as a result of tissue edema (**Fig. 10.7.1**). This enhancement was absent from the patient's right breast. The examination detected pathological lymph nodes in the left axilla.

Ultrasonographic examination showed a large tumor mass rich in vessels (**Fig. 10.7.2**). Ultrasound-guided core biopsy was performed and proved malignancy as well as the invasive character of the cancer (**Fig. 10.7.3**, CAM 5.2 immunostaining).

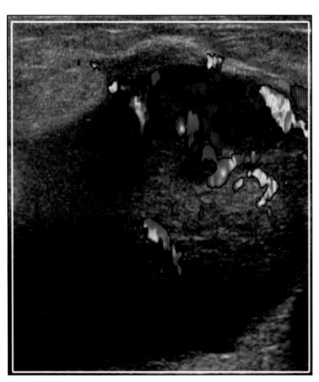

Fig. 10.7.2

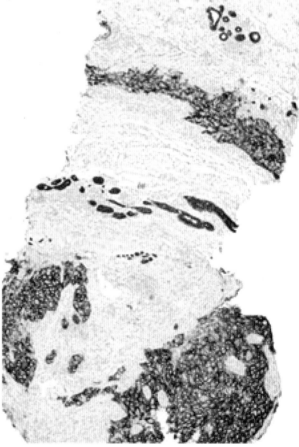

Fig. 10.7.3

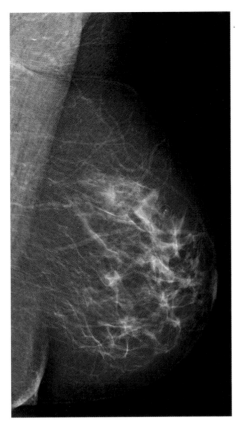

Fig. 10.7.4

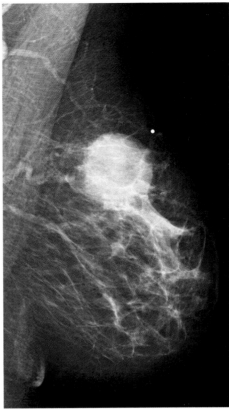

Fig. 10.7.5

The breast tissue was almost completely involuted (fatty involution, Tabár pattern II) and the mammograms were easy to read. No abnormality could be detected on the mammogram shown in **Fig. 10.7.4** taken 6 months prior to the detection of the palpable lump. The tumor was easy to perceive on the mammogram at the time of presentation (**Fig. 10.7.5**). Immunohistochemistry of the core biopsy specimen showed a very high proliferative activity of the tumor cells (**Fig. 10.7.6**, Ki67 immunostaining), explaining the rapid growth of the tumor, and also indicated the sensitivity of the tumor cells for cytotoxic agents.

The patient underwent preoperative (neoadjuvant) chemotherapy. The mammogram taken after treatment (**Fig. 10.7.7**) demonstrated a very good response because the tumor had practically disappeared.

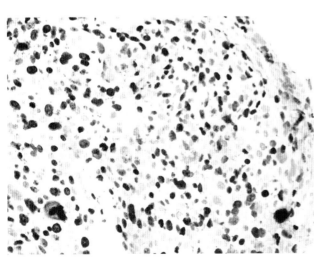

Fig. 10.7.6

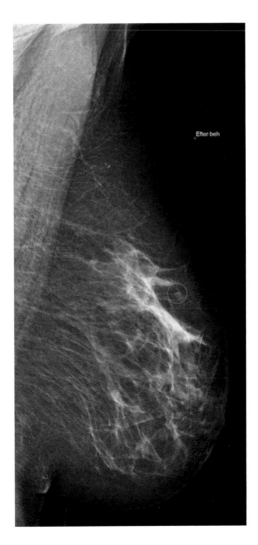

Fig. 10.7.7

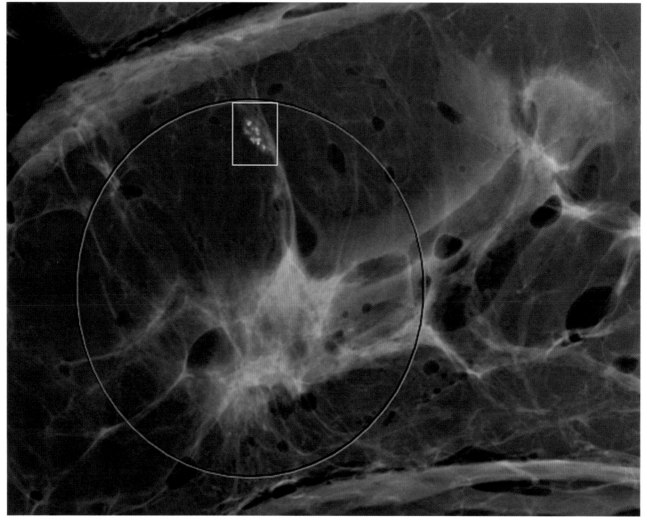

Fig. 10.7.8

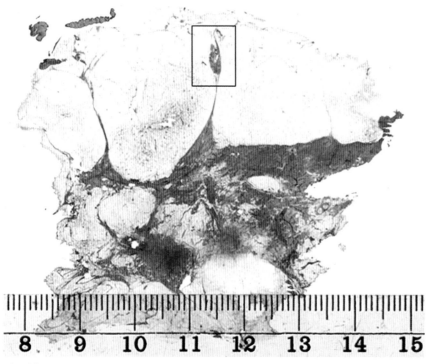

Fig. 10.7.9

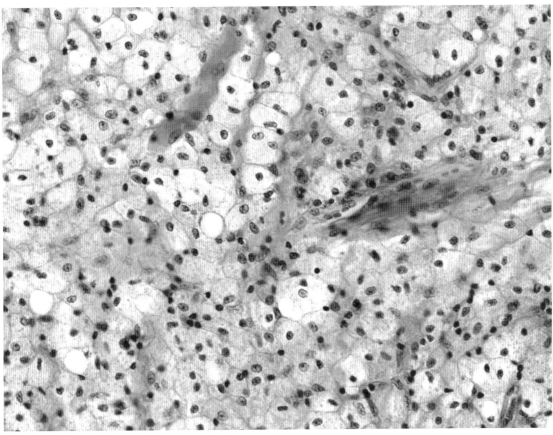

Fig. 10.7.10

Mastectomy and axillary clearance were performed after the neoadjuvant chemotherapy was completed. **Figs. 10.7.8** and **10.7.10** are a mastectomy specimen slice radiographs showing an exceptionally good response. The slice of the mastectomy specimen demonstrated in **Fig. 10.7.8** contained a small calcified fibroadenoma, which was easily identified in both the radiogram and the corresponding large-format histology slide (marked in **Figs. 10.7.8** and **10.7.9**). Thorough histological analysis of several large sections from the specimen revealed areas of inflammation, necrosis, infiltrates of histiocytes (**Fig.10.7.11**), and widespread serous edema of the fatty tissue, but no viable cancer cells were found.

Fig. 10.7.11

Conclusions

Highly proliferative breast carcinomas are usually sensitive to chemotherapy. Neoadjuvant chemotherapy may lead to complete remission of such tumors. Detailed histological examination is necessary to assess the effect of such therapeutic intervention.

Case 8. "Basal-like" Breast Cancer

This 66-year-old woman felt a lump in her left breast. She had undergone a screening mammography examination 13 months earlier, which showed a tiny lesion that had not been perceived (**Fig. 10.8.1**). A comparison of the previous and current mammograms (**Figs. 10.8.1** and **10.8.2**) illustrates the rapid growth of the tumor.

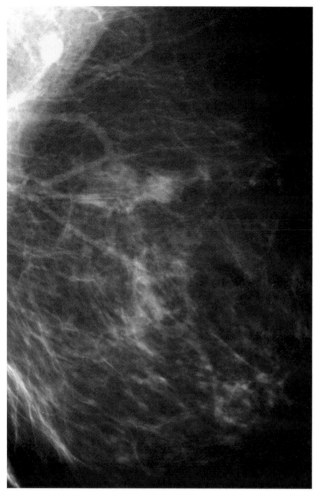

Fig. 10.8.1

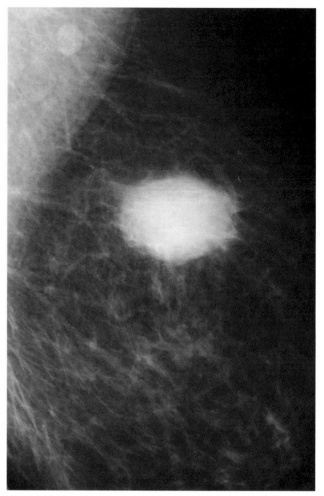

Fig. 10.8.2

The tumor presented as a solitary oval mass on the mammogram (**Fig. 10.8.2**) and on breast ultrasound. (**Fig. 10.8.3**) and measured 33 × 24 mm. It showed so-called rim enhancement on magnetic resonance imaging (**Fig. 10.8.4**) typical of centrally necrotic or fibrotic rapidly growing tumors. The radiological appearance of the tumor correlated well with that in the large-format histology slide (**Fig. 10.8.5**, in which the cranial and the nipple margins are marked).

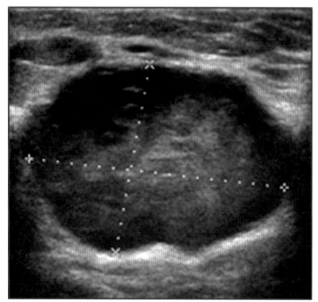

Fig. 10.8.3

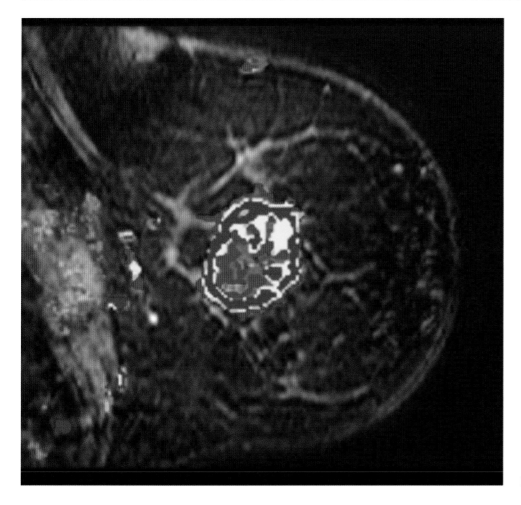

Fig. 10.8.4

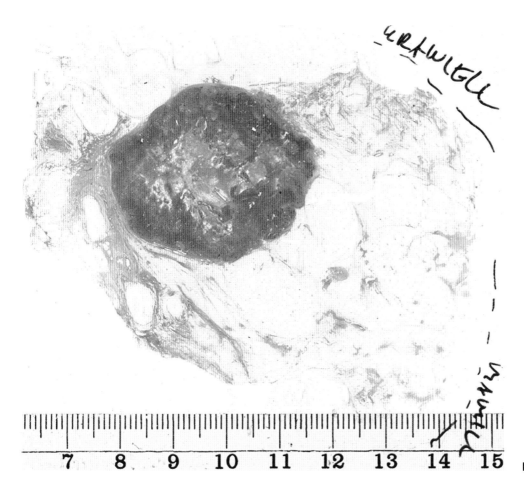

Fig. 10.8.5

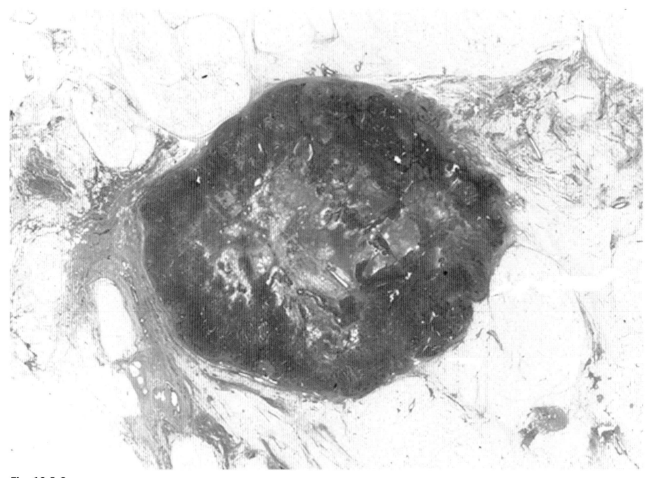

Fig. 10.8.6

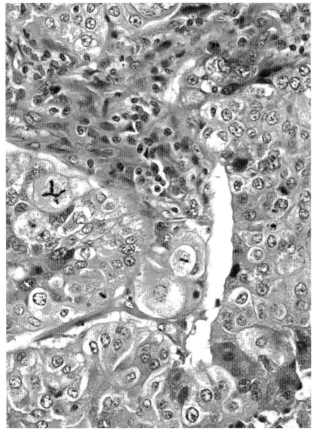

Fig. 10.8.7

Detailed histological examination showed a unifocal, 40 × 34-mm, grade III, invasive ductal carcinoma (**Fig. 10.8.6**) without a demonstrable in situ component. The tumor cells were atypical and showed high mitotic activity. Atypical mitotic figures were also present (**Fig. 10.8.7**). A moderately dense lymphocytic infiltrate was present in the stroma of the tumor. Vascular invasion was not seen, and the two examined axillary sentinel lymph nodes were free of cancer cells.

Immunohistochemical phenotyping of the tumor revealed that the tumor cells neither expressed estrogen or progesterone receptors nor HER-2. High proliferative activity was detected in the tumor with Ki67 immunostaining. Most of the tumor cells expressed cytokeratin 5/6 and cytokeratin 14 typical of the myoepithelium of the normal breast (**Fig. 10.8.8**). The tumor also showed focal epithelial growth factor receptor (EGFR) positivity (**10.8.9**). Thus the tumor was classified as triple-negative basal-like cancer.

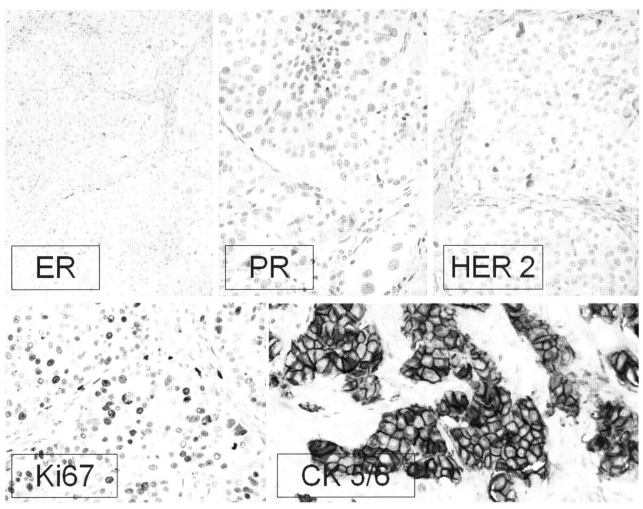

Fig. 10.8.8

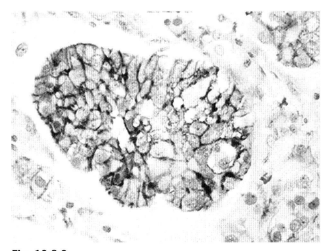

Fig. 10.8.9

Conclusions

Basal-like breast carcinomas represent a heterogeneous group of tumors, many of which are rapidly growing round/ oval masses showing central necrosis. Proper classification of such tumors requires routine use of a panel of antibodies for immunohistochemical characterization of the tumor cells.
As mentioned in Chapter 9, although the clinical importance of expression of myoepithelial markers by the cancer cells is increasingly evident, there is still no international consensus on the definition of basal-like cancers.

Case 9. Multifocal Invasive Carcinoma

This 49-year-old woman felt a lump under her right areola. A slight skin retraction could be provoked over the tumor. Physical examination confirmed the presence of a hard tumor and revealed a "thickening" in the upper and central portions of the right breast.

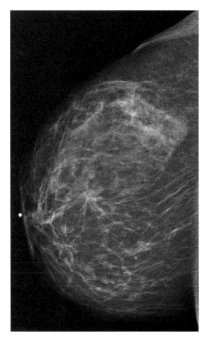

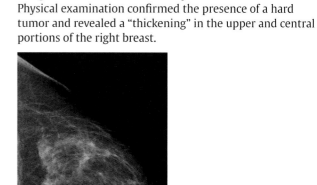

Fig. 10.9.1

Fig. 10.9.2

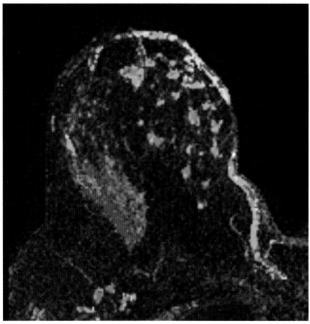

Fig. 10.9.3

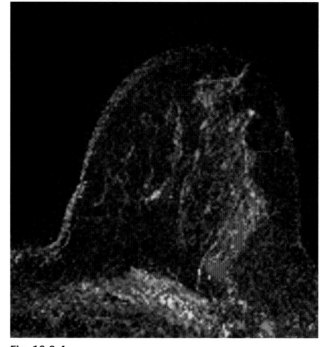

Fig. 10.9.4

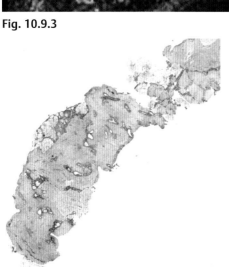

Fig. 10.9.5

Mammography (Fig. 10.9.1) and magnetic resonance imaging (Fig. 10.9.3) demonstrated at least 30 individual tumor foci with washout pattern in her right breast. Pathological lymph nodes were detected in the right axilla.

The nonpalpable lesion in her left breast (Figs. 10.9.2 and 10.9.4) was a benign fibroadenoma at core biopsy (Fig. 10.9.5).

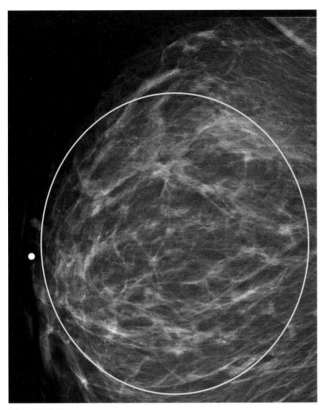

Fig. 10.9.6

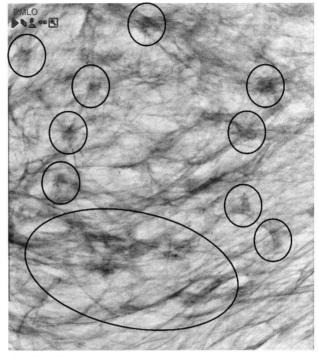

Fig. 10.9.7

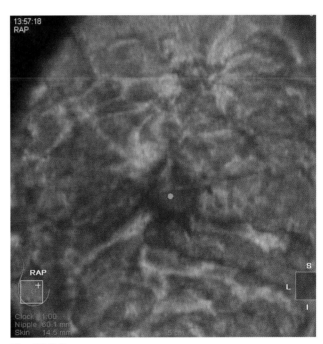

Fig. 10.9.8

The multiple tumor foci were easily perceived on microfocus magnification radiographs (**Figs. 10.9.6** and **10.9.7**, digitally inverted image) and on three-dimensional automated ultrasonographic examination (**Fig. 10.9.8**). All of the four ultrasound-guided core biopsies from the most distant foci contained invasive cancer, proving the multifocal nature of the disease (**Fig. 10.9.9**). The largest focus measured 14 mm on magnetic resonance imaging. The radiologically measured disease extent was 100 × 60 × 59 mm.

The examination was completed with fine-needle aspiration of a pathological lymph node from the right axilla revealing malignant cells.

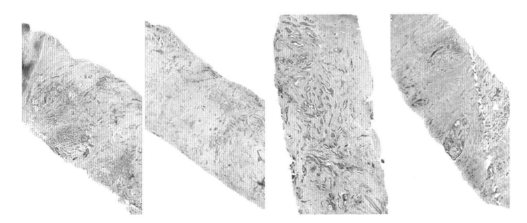

Fig. 10.9.9

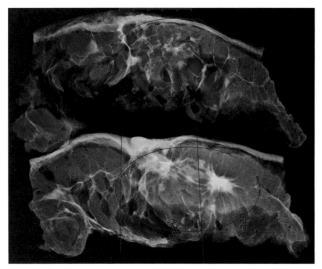

Fig. 10.9.10

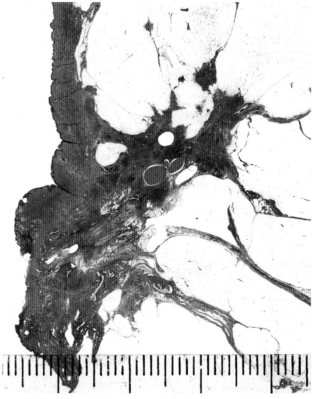

Fig. 10.9.11

Large-format histology sections from the mastectomy specimen demonstrated more than 25 individual foci of invasive ductal carcinoma grade II, the largest focus measuring 33 × 15 mm and the smallest 1 mm. Foci of in situ carcinoma were also seen. There was a very good correlation between the preoperative imaging findings, specimen radiographs, radiographs of the sliced specimen (**Figs. 10.9.10** and **10.9.13**), and the findings in large-format histology slides. The large sections in **Figs. 10.9.11** and **10.9.14** demonstrate the histological extent of the disease (~ 80 × 70 mm) and also reveal involvement of the nipple and the skin of the areola (**Fig. 10.9.11**).

The invasive component of the tumor was of Luminal A phenotype and expressed estrogen (**Fig. 10.9.12**) and progesterone receptors but not HER2. The Ki67 proliferation index was low. However, vascular invasion was evident and 6 out of the 17 examined axillary lymph nodes contained macrometastatic deposits (**Fig. 10.9.15**). The largest deposit measured 11 mm.

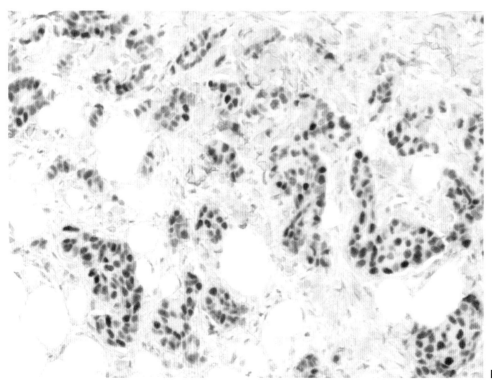

Fig. 10.9.12

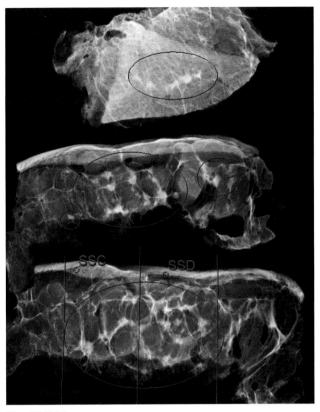

Fig. 10.9.13

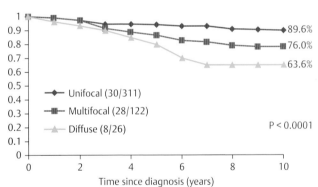

Fig. 10.9.14

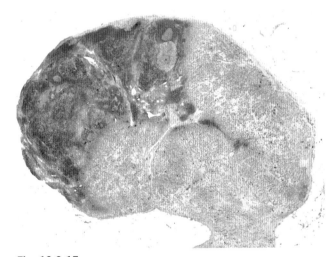

Fig. 10.9.15

Fig. 10.9.16 Cumulative disease-specific survival in 459 consecutive breast carcinoma cases by distribution of the invasive component. Dalarna County, 1996–1998. (Reproduced with permission of the publisher, the same as Fig. 9.18.)

Conclusions

Multifocality of the invasive component of breast carcinoma is associated with a high risk of metastatic spread of the tumor cells to the lymph nodes. The metastases are most often macrometastases (> 2 mm in size). Multifocality is also associated with poorer survival of the patients compared to those having unifocal tumors (**Fig. 10.9.16**).

Case 10. Breast Carcinoma with Diffuse In Situ and Multifocal Invasive Component: A Lobar Disease

This 39-year-old woman felt a thickening in her left breast. The mammograms showed a large breast lobe filled with microcalcifications of the casting type; an entire quadrant of the left breast was involved (**Figs. 10.10.1, 10.10.2,** and **10.10.3**).

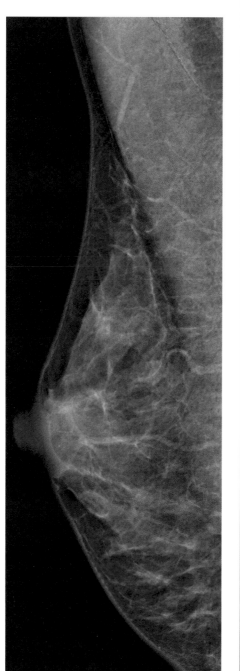

Fig. 10.10.1

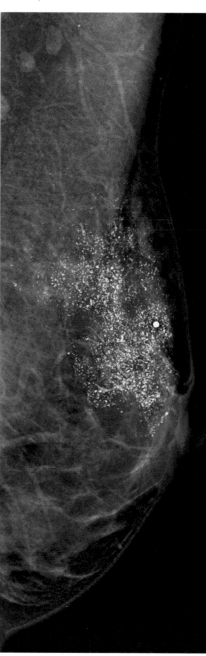

Fig. 10.10.2

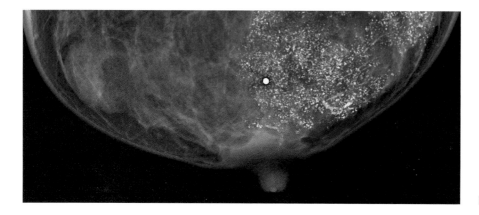

Fig. 10.10.3

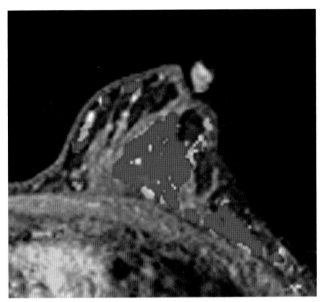

Fig. 10.10.4

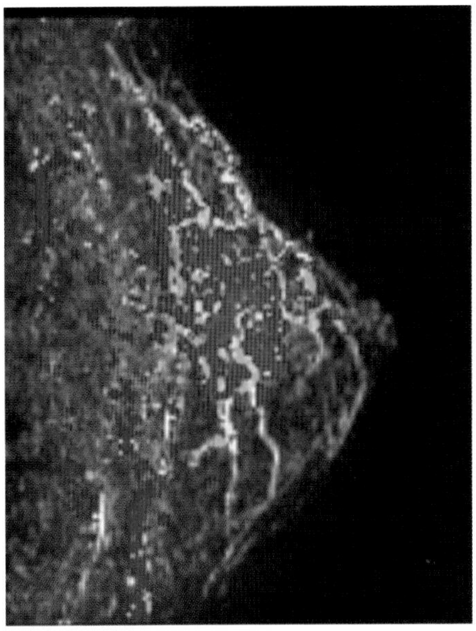

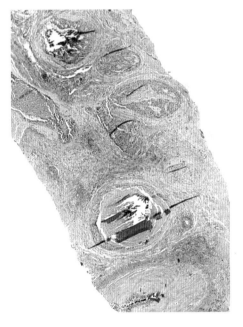

Fig. 10.10.5

Magnetic resonance imaging revealed a diffuse-segmental contrast enhancement corresponding to the involved lobe (**Figs. 10.10.4** and **10.10.5**).

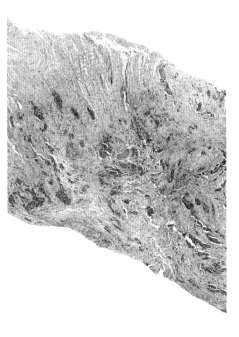

Fig. 10.10.7

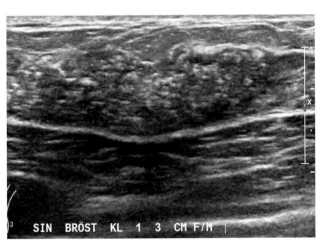

Fig. 10.10.6

Handheld ultrasound-guided core biopsies from different parts of the lesion contained structures of both in situ and invasive cancer (**Figs. 10.10.6**, **10.10.7**, and **10.10.8**).

Fig. 10.10.8

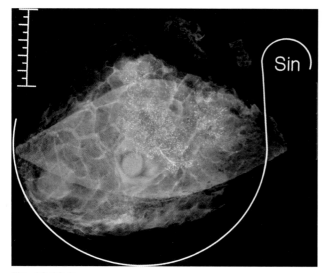

Fig. 10.10.9

Mastectomy and sentinel lymph node biopsy were performed. The specimen radiograph (**Fig. 10.10.9**) shows the lobar distribution of microcalcifications and the extensive nature of the lesion. **Fig. 10.10.11** represents a tissue slice reconstructed from five adjacent large-format histology sections and is compared with the radiograph of the same tissue slice in **Fig. 10.10.10**. The histological extent of the disease is marked and measured 95 × 70 mm.

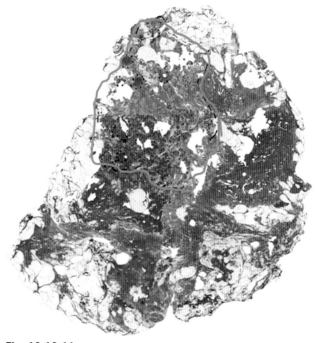

Fig. 10.10.11

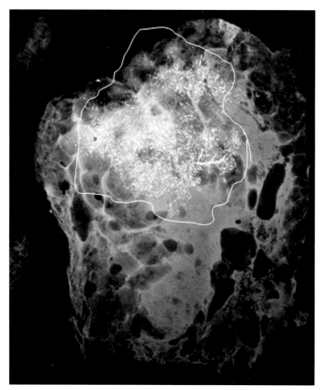

Fig. 10.10.10

In addition to the extensive in situ component, the tumor contained seven separate invasive foci (encircled in **Fig. 10.10.12**) measuring 5 to 10 mm in their largest dimension.

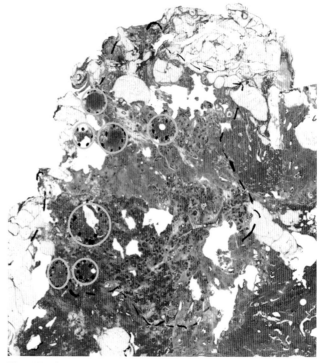

Fig. 10.10.12

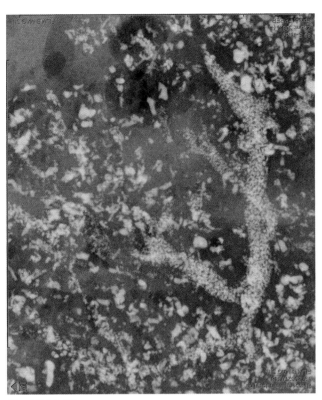

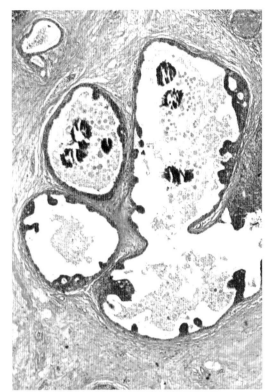

Fig. 10.10.13

Fig. 10.10.14

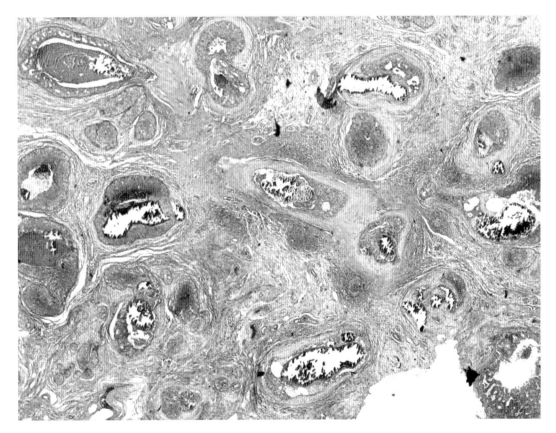

Fig. 10.10.15

On microfocus magnification of the specimen radiograph two types of calcifications were distinguished: dotted casting-type calcifications resembling the skin of a snake (in the branching duct in the right half in **Fig. 10.10.13**) and fragmented casting-type calcifications.

Dotted casting-type calcifications were found in ducts and ductlike structures containing the elements of micropapillary DCIS (**Fig.10.10.14**), whereas fragmented casting-type microcalcifications were present in the solid part of the DCIS component of the tumor (**Fig. 10.10.15**).

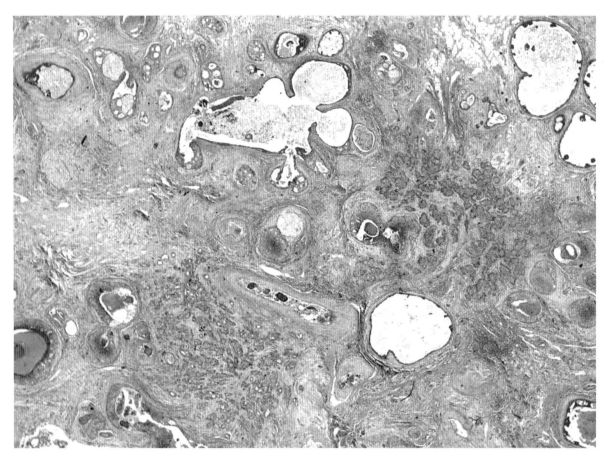

Fig. 10.10.16

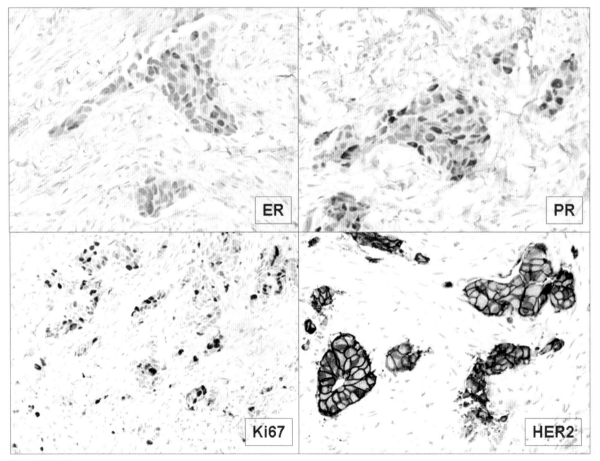

Fig. 10.10.17

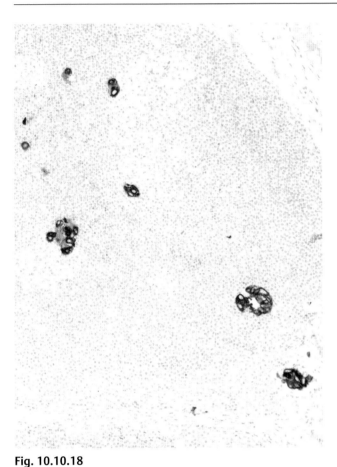

The invasive foci of the tumor represented grade II ductal carcinomas (**Fig. 10.10.16**) expressing estrogen and progesterone receptors and HER-2. The Ki67 proliferation index was 15%, indicating an intermediate proliferative activity of the tumor cells in the invasive component (**Fig. 10.10.17**). Dispersed tumor cell groups were found in one of the two examined axillary sentinel lymph nodes (**Fig. 10.10.18**, CAM 5.2 immunostaining).

A close look at the mammogram of the nipple revealed the presence of microcalcifications in the lactiferous duct of the involved lobe and in its branches (**Fig. 10.10.19**), indicating the lobar nature of the disease.

Conclusions

The lobar nature of breast carcinoma is best perceived in tumors having an extensive diffuse (usually high-grade) in situ component.

Fig. 10.10.18

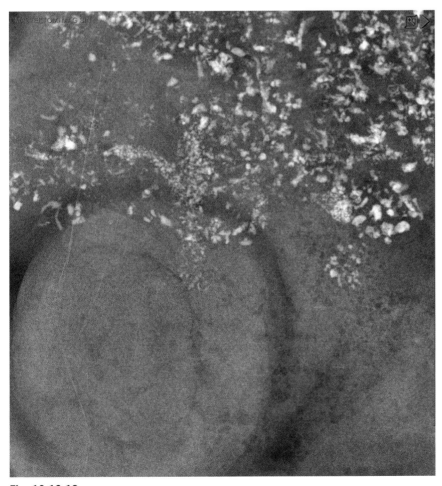

Fig. 10.10.19

Index